Praise for
*How to Manage Nursing Care at Home*

**By Douglas Winslow Cooper, Ph.D., and Diane R. Beggin, R.N.**

As a 20-year caregiver for my wife, father, and grandmother, one of my main challenges has been getting accurate and thorough information about home care. Dr. Cooper's herculean efforts to provide a quality life for both his wife and mother, even as they lost all mobility and the ability to communicate, provide both inspiration and a wealth of information for America's millions of caretakers.

**J. Steve Miller, co-author of *Why Brilliant People Believe Nonsense* and author of *Faith That Is Not Blind,* professor, caregiver**

*How to Manage Nursing Care at Home* delivers an extraordinary account of home care practices and goes in tandem with my book *The Ultimate Compassionate Guide to Caregiving.* These are excellent resources for caring for your loved ones in the home.

**Tena L. Scallan owner of http://www.theultimatecaregivingexpert. com, a new and innovative blog that provides education and advice on all aspects of caregiving for caregivers and their families**

"...authors Douglas Winslow Cooper and Diane R. Beggin address one of the most complex global issues faced in the 21st century: caring for someone you love, one who is also diagnosed with a severe medical condition, doing this safely, and in the home.... a valuable guide that will ease your worry as you begin your journey as one of the millions of untrained family caregivers who want to safely provide complex medical care services so that your loved one can remain home."

**From the Foreword by Eboni I. Green, PhD, RN, Co-Founder of Caregiver Support Services, www.caregiversupportservices.org**

꩜꩜꩜

This book is a total comprehensive guide for any family choosing complete care at home for seriously ill family members. Well thought out, clear, it has detailed information relating to every area needing attention. A "must read" handbook for family members and caregivers alike!

**Lauri Privett, President, Personally Delivered Home Health & Incontinence Products**

꩜꩜꩜

Cooper and Beggin have packed their book chock-full of useful information—it is complete, comprehensive, and well thought-out.

Readers of *How to Manage Nursing Care at Home* will also find a detailed list of recommended equipment and supplies to make their jobs easier, an explanation of human body functions (to help them better understand what their loved one is going through), care considerations for different conditions, advice on hiring qualified nursing help, and sample paperwork you can use to oversee that nursing help (instead of the other way around).

As our country's population continues to age, information for prospective, new, and current caregivers will become king. The information shared in *How to Manage Nursing Care at Home* can prove to be and will prove to be a valuable read for anybody stepping into the role of a family caregiver or already serving as one for a loved one with a chronic health condition not living in a long-term care home.

**Rick Lauber—Author of *Caregiver's Guide for Canadians and The Successful Caregiver's Guide***

# HOW TO MANAGE
# *Nursing Care*
# AT HOME

*Deciding on, Preparing for,
and Managing Home Care*

Douglas Winslow Cooper, Ph.D.
Diane R. Beggin, R.N.

outskirts
press

# DEDICATION

*For those who take on the difficult and generous task of caring for their patients in the context of the family home.*

*In memory of Diana Winslow Cooper, LPN, who cared deeply and well for all her patients and for her family and was, in return, much loved, and in memory of our dear mother, Priscilla Taylor Cooper, also greatly loved.*

*In memory of Donald J. Steinbrenner, Diane Beggin's beloved twin brother. Don died much too young from consequences of hemophilia. His death, but foremost his perseverance in living with a chronic disease, and the birth of her hemophiliac son helped kindle Diane's interest in medicine and nursing.*

*And in memory of our colleague Angela J. Mullins, LPN, whose skilled care, humor, and great personal warmth have been greatly missed, due to her tragically early death.*

# ACKNOWLEDGMENTS

We appreciate the help we have gotten from the doctors and nurses involved in our own situation of providing nursing care at home and, most recently, in the writing of this book. We thank the following:

**Drs. A. Baradaran, P. Chidyllo, A. Fruchter, F. Guneratne, S. Koyfman, R. F. Walker,** and the doctors and nurses at Orange Regional Medical Center, Middletown, NY, who have given the care that has helped preserve our patients' lives.

**Cheryl C. Cohen** for her friendship, encouragement, and editorial aid.

**Eboni Ivory Green, PhD, RN** for sharing her medical and editorial expertise and for contributing to our book her Foreword and Appendix 1 on tips for caregivers.

**Adria Goldman Gross** for her friendship and generous sharing of portions of our co-authored book, *SOLVED! Curing Your Medical Insurance Problems*.

**IBM,** for their continuing generous support for the past twelve years for skilled nursing care at home of our beloved Tina S. Cooper.

**Rick Lauber,** for his encouraging comments, and his highly informative *The Successful Caregiver's Guide.*

**Ellen Puleo, LPN,** for her skilled nursing help and her editorial aid, and for their helpful comments: **Luanne Furman, RN; Annamarie Carotenuto-Odland, RN;** and **Maureen McDermott, RN, BA, MA, CCRN.**

**Tena L. Scallan,** for her supportive words and her encyclopedic *The Ultimate Compassionate Guide to Caregiving.*

# PREFACE

**According to AARP (2015), 16.6%, one out of every six, of Americans provide unpaid care to an adult. In many cases, this care goes beyond custodial care and qualifies as skilled nursing care.**

We wrote this book to make it easier for those who step forward to provide care in their home for a family member or friend, although not being trained medical professionals themselves. One can manage something without being an expert, but it does require a working knowledge of the major concepts and implementation of some variety of systematization. Whether you are managing the care at home or just monitoring care being given at home by an agency, this book should be of assistance to you in understanding what is needed and what is being done.

**Having managed nursing care at home for my wife**, bedridden with multiple sclerosis for over two decades, with around-the-clock skilled nursing for the past twelve years, involving ventilator use and gastric tube feeding and medicating, I [DWC] decided to prepare this book, with our head nurse [DRB], to help others succeed in managing or monitoring nursing care at home, for themselves and their loved ones.

**Diane R. Beggin, RN**, became our head nurse soon after starting with us in 2004, and she has developed many of the systems and documents we have used to care for my wife and also, for the past several years, to care for my bedridden, nearly-100-year-old mother, Priscilla Taylor Cooper, who died in November of 2015.

*How to Manage Nursing Care at Home* tells its readers what to expect and gives them the necessary information and structure, in terms of needed forms, "charts," to understand and oversee the nursing care given by RNs and LPNs.

We invite our readers to contact us with their questions and with recommendations for our subsequent publications on providing nursing care at home.

**Douglas Winslow Cooper, PhD**
264 East Drive, Walden, NY 12586
douglas@tingandi.com

**Diane R. Beggin, RN**
40 Sycamore Drive, Montgomery, NY 12549
DianeBegginRN@gmail.com

# DISCLAIMER

This publication does not offer advice on the medical treatment of patients, which is the appropriate task for specially trained medical professionals having detailed knowledge of the patient. It is intended to assist the intelligent layman in managing nursing care in the home.

Although this is the product of our experience and diligent research, we assume no liability for the information provided here. Use of this work releases us from any loss or other liability incurred by the user.

# FOREWORD

*"Let whoever is in charge keep this simple question in her head: not, how can I always do this right thing myself, but how can I provide for this right thing to be always done?"*
Florence Nightingale[1]

Emperor Marcus Aurelius is one of my favorite authors. Living during a time when the world was constantly at war, disease was rampant, and there was a great deal of human suffering, the Emperor, a stoic, believed in self-restraint. He also lived with the knowledge that the decisions he made would impact the lives of millions of people.

Marcus Aurelius firmly believed that wisdom was obtained by examining oneself, so he took time to journal his private thoughts each night as a method of personal improvement. His philosophical reflections were never intended to be shared with the public; rather, they were his true and visceral responses to what he was experiencing, and a free expression of frustrations associated with the challenges he faced daily as a person with many flaws.

His once-private meditations continue to be relevant to coping with challenges we humans encounter two thousand years later. Marcus Aurelius did not set out to be an author, yet his published works highlight the importance of sharing your wisdom.

---

1    Florence Nightingale. Retrieved on October 17, 2016 from http://www.goodreads.com/author/quotes/63031.Florence_Nightingale

In *How to Manage Nursing Care at Home*, authors Douglas Winslow Cooper and Diane R. Beggin, address one of the most complex global issues faced in the 21st century: caring for someone you love, one who is also diagnosed with a severe medical condition, doing this safely, and in the home.

The truth is that there is no easy way to address the immense fiscal and logistical barriers that must be considered as you take on the responsibility for providing nursing-level care at home. I can personally attest to the challenges associated with ensuring that a loved one safely receives full-time complex medical care–24 hours a day, seven days a week–for an indefinite period of time.

As a registered nurse and the co-founder of Caregiver Support Services, a non-profit organization that exists to improve the health and wellbeing of both family and professional caregivers, I have dedicated my life to improving the circumstances of the elderly and their caregivers.

I am also a caregiver for my mother-in-law, Emma. Earlier this year, she was infected with a virulent strain of influenza, was placed on a ventilator, went into a medically induced coma, and suffered a stroke. We didn't know if she would survive. Mom has since transitioned to a rehabilitation center to receive therapy, but our goal is to bring her home.

A major barrier to Mom's transition to home is coordinating the complex care that she needs. One of our biggest concerns is that Mom wakes up three or more times each night to urinate, but she can't remember that she is unable to walk to the bathroom safely on her own. So, when she tries to stand up from bed, she often falls. In fact, my husband and I receive a call from the rehab center once or twice a week reporting that Mom has fallen. This repetitive circumstance is heartbreaking.

Waking up multiple times a night has led to decreased daytime functioning for Mom, and even more concerning, to anxiety and depression. These additional issues have made it extremely challenging to engage her in the recovery therapies necessary for her to return home. In fact, we meet regularly with the staff and the doctors to modify her anxiety and depression medications to help her achieve the highest level of functioning.

We want to bring Mom home, but we are physically and emotionally overwhelmed. Our biggest concern is pulling together everything needed to make the transition safely. In fact, just the thought of trying to figure out where to start to gather the resources that we will need to bring her home has been downright stressful. This book addresses such issues.

Dr. Cooper includes firsthand experiences associated with caring for his wife, Tina, who is quadriplegic, on a ventilator, and suffers from multiple sclerosis. Together they have overcome tremendous obstacles, yet because of Dr. Cooper's advocacy and with the help of her head nurse, Diane R. Beggin, Tina is lovingly being cared for in her home.

What likely began as a way to cope and to document his very personal experience with caring for Tina has been nurtured and is now a valuable guide that will ease your worry as you begin your journey as one of the millions of untrained family caregivers who want to safely provide complex medical care services so that your loved one can remain home.

I know that this text has helped my family with starting the process to bring Mom home. In fact, these distinguished authors go a step further than most books written about caregiving, as they address both the emotional and navigational aspects of caring for someone you love.

I am honored to have gotten to know Tina, Dr. Cooper, and Tina's nurse, Diane Beggin, through reading their very personal experience of providing complex care in the home. Like Marcus Aurelius, the authors of this important work have openly shared their wisdom so that you do not have to face the immense challenges associated with caregiving alone.

I leave you with this final thought,

> *Knowledge comes, but wisdom lingers. It may not be difficult to store up in the mind a vast quantity of facts within a comparatively short time, but the ability to form judgments requires the severe discipline of hard work and the tempering heat of experience and maturity.*[2]

The care of your loved one will require planning and the continuous acquisition of knowledge to ensure all needs are being met, including your own. Juggling all of the challenges will likely be difficult, yet this useful contribution to caregiving highlights your intangible contributions as a part of the healthcare infrastructure.

I hope that you will take advantage of the wisdom shared in the pages that follow, that you are empowered to use this material

---

2    Calvin Coolidge. BrainyQuote.com, Xplore Inc., 2016. https://www.brainyquote.com/quotes/quotes/c/calvincool156506.html, accessed October 24, 2016.

to make your life easier, and that you continue to seek additional learning opportunities as your caregiving situation changes.

Eboni I. Green, PhD, RN
Co-Founder of Caregiver Support Services
www.caregiversupportservices.org

# TABLE OF CONTENTS

# INTRODUCTION

Our book should be of help to those who want to set up nursing care at home for a patient coming directly from the hospital or from a nursing home or rehabilitation facility that has served as an intermediate step. The patient has a severe and possibly chronic medical condition requiring skilled nursing care.

Basically, your choices are carrying out nursing care at home or putting the individual into a facility already set up to provide nursing care, such as a hospice, a nursing home, a long-term-care facility, but probably not an assisted-living community, as we are assuming that skilled nursing care will be required. We describe what we have learned by caring for two patients at home and what we have gleaned from our other experience and from the medical and nursing literature.

## NURSING CARE AT HOME

"In the United States, about 40 million people provide unpaid care to an ill or disabled adult. One quarter of those caregivers have been in their roles for five years or longer. And these loving helpers often go it alone. Only half of family caregivers say they get unpaid help from another family member or friend." (AARP, 2015)

Nursing care at home can range from around-the-clock nursing for someone with a critical condition to regular or even intermittent visits by a nurse to care for someone who continues to live in the home almost exclusively.

**Many people would prefer for themselves or their loved ones the option of nursing care at home rather than having to go live in a separate facility.** Depending on the particular details of the situation, this can be significantly more, but sometimes less, expensive than being in a nursing facility. This option requires management, the primary focus of this book.

## PROBLEMS

The patient in question is being released from the hospital under the condition that the next stop is either a nursing home, a hospice, or a suitably equipped home, yours. You have decided to take on the responsibility of having the patient at home. Now what?

## SOLUTIONS

We will show you **how to plan** for the patient's homecoming, select **where** the patient will be cared for, and determine **who** will provide **what** care **when,** and **how** and **with what** equipment and material.

## THE AUTHORS

**Douglas Winslow Cooper, PhD,** is a writer, editor, and retired environmental scientist, who **for over a decade has helped to manage continuous, at-home, skilled nursing care of his wife, Tina Su Cooper, quadriplegic and ventilator-dependent due to multiple sclerosis.** For several years, he also managed the skilled nursing care at home of his nearly-100-year-old mother, bedridden, virtually quadriplegic, ventilator-dependent, medicated and fed through a gastric tube, and on a pacemaker.

Douglas earned his A.B., with honors, in physics at Cornell, served at the U.S. Army biological warfare laboratories at Ft. Detrick, MD, returned to school and obtained his M.S. degree in physics at Penn State and his Ph.D. in engineering from Harvard. His professional life centered on environmental issues.

He served as an Associate Professor at the Harvard Graduate School of Public Health, was Director of the Environmental Health Management Program, and subsequently conducted environmental studies as a Research Staff Member at IBM's Yorktown Heights, NY, Thomas J. Watson, Jr., Research Center.

**Dr. Cooper was the author or co-author of more than 100 technical articles published in refereed journals and was elected Fellow of the Institute of Environmental Sciences. He now does freelance writing, book coaching/partnering, and editing.** He wrote *Ting and I: A Memoir of Love, Courage, and Devotion,* co-authored three other memoirs, coached for and edited three other non-fiction books. Most recently, he co-authored *SOLVED! Curing Your Medical Insurance Problems,* and *Frustrated with Life? You Are Not Alone!* and wrote *Write Your Book with Me.* He continues to work with would-be authors.

Contact information:
Douglas Winslow Cooper, PhD, LLC
264 East Drive, Walden, NY
douglas@tingandi.com
http://ManageNursingCareAtHome.com

**Diane R. Beggin, RN:** Originally hoping to become a veterinarian, but unable to finance achieving that goal, Diane R. Beggin's earliest professional career was in the financial industry. She started working in a Dean Witter Reynolds branch office (now Morgan Stanley) in California and **later transferred to the World Trade Center in New York, where she became a vice-president in operations.** While a manager, she found that organizational skills and development of intra-departmental documentation proved vital.

**Diane "retired" from this successful career to raise a family. When her children were young, she returned to school for a career in nursing. After graduating with her RN from Orange County Community College (SUNY Orange), winning the Spirit of Nursing Award from the Army Nurse Corps, and being recognized for her officer roles in the Nursing Club and Phi Theta Kappa, Diane began her career as a Professional Registered Nurse [RN] directly in the critical care unit.**

A disabling injury prevented her from continuing in hospital-based nursing. Soon afterward, in the fall of 2004, Diane began working for Dr. Cooper to assist in the skilled nursing care in their home of his wife, who was expected to survive only a few months, but who has survived for twelve more years.

Over these past twelve years, Diane has continued to work both part-time for the Coopers and in other nursing venues. **Diane, as head nurse for Dr. Cooper, has used her training and experience to establish the documentation and protocols used in the daily practice of caring for two quadriplegic, ventilator–dependent patients in the home.** She also completes the quarterly physician orders and extensive semi-annual insurance reports detailing the clinical status for Mrs. Tina Cooper to justify her continued medical insurance benefits.

**Diane Beggin has collaborated in the preparation and writing of this book in hopes that it will prove of value to others seeking to manage nursing care in the home. She is currently available for consulting on such matters.**

Contact information:
Diane R. Beggin, RN
40 Sycamore Drive
Montgomery, NY 12549
DianeBegginRN@gmail.com
http://managenursingcareathome.com

## WHAT YOU WILL LEARN

**Why choose home care** rather than care at a nursing facility?
**Where** in your home?
**What** will you need?
**When** will who have to do what?
**Whom** will you hire?
**How** will you manage the care?

## OUR PROMISE

**You will learn from our experience** how to prepare for the homecoming of your patient and how to manage nursing care at home thereafter.

## YOUR OPPORTUNITY AND RESPONSIBILITY

Providing skilled nursing care at home is both challenging and rewarding for the caregivers. **Home care is a blessing for the patient.** Having chosen to provide it, you deserve to congratulate yourself. To make this project more manageable, take advantage of the advice and the forms provided here.

## HOME FROM THE HOSPITAL

Someone you care deeply about is being released from the hospital, with the alternatives of home care, hospice care, or a nursing home. You have to decide, or help them decide, which alternative is best. If you decide on home care, you may need to manage it. This book will help you understand how to provide skilled nursing care at home and will aid in your decision-making.

**As noted, the co-authors have been involved for over a decade in supplying and managing skilled nursing care at home** for Tina Su Cooper (Cooper, 2011):

*In June of 2004, when she came home from the Critical Care Unit after the 100 days that nearly killed her, Tina was on a ventilator, quadriplegic, fed through a gastric tube. Not only was she totally dependent on us for her care, the list of infections and problems that had developed while hospitalized was daunting. She had been "colonized" by two strains of hospital-acquired bacteria and given only months to live. She was safer at home or in a hospice than in the hospital, our doctors agreed. Being given the choice of home or the hospice meant there was a good chance she had only months to live. She took it in stride.*

**Over a decade later, Tina's health has remained strong,** and even though the losses caused by multiple sclerosis have been severe, including quadriplegia, dependence on a ventilator and the need to be fed and medicated by a gastric tube, she has been able to live an added thirteen years and generally enjoys her life at home.

We, the co-authors, have long thought it worthwhile to write a book about our experience, but only recently got down to doing it. **Investigating what was available at mega-bookseller amazon.com, we found only one relevant entry when we queried "manage nursing care at home."** That book, *How to Manage Family Illness at Home*, which we will describe next, was written by a British author, Gill Pharaoh, published in paperback in 2004, re-issued as a Kindle e-book in 2015.

The chapter list for Ms. Pharaoh's book is as follows:

Chapter 1: Receiving the Diagnosis
Chapter 2: Whom to Tell?
Chapter 3: The Services of the Hospice and Palliative Care Team
Chapter 4: Making Decisions about Work
Chapter 5: How Much to Tell the Children?
Chapter 6: Caring for the Carer
Chapter 7: Looking at Ways in Which Everyone Can Help
Chapter 8: The Physical Needs of the Person Who is Ill*
Chapter 9: The Use of Aids and Appliances*
Chapter 10: Some Common Symptoms and the Use of Medication
Chapter 11: Physical Comfort, Health, and Safety for Everyone Involved

**Ms. Pharaoh's valuable book emphasizes the many significant psycho-social aspects of home care, and hospice care at home, two areas we are not going to explore in depth.** Her two chapters that we have marked with asterisks cover topics similar to what is covered here, where we go into the "nuts and bolts" of managing nursing care for someone at home.

**A less restrictive search, for ebooks covering "nursing care at home," gave the following titles:**

- *Long Term Care: Everything You Need to Know about Long Term Care Nursing and How to Plan and Pay for Long Term Care and Insurance [2014]*
- *Nursing Wild Birds for Release at Home: Booklet [2014]*
- *Now and at the Hour of Our Death [2015]*
- *American Cancer Society Complete Guide to Family Caregiving: the Essential Guide to Cancer Caregiving at Home [2012]*
- *Keeping Your Mind While They're Losing Theirs: a*

*Sometimes Poignant Look at Dealing with a Parent who Has Alzheimer's or Dementia [2015]*
- *Five Ways to Pay for Home Healthcare and Stay in Your Home [2012]*
- *AIDS Care at Home: A Guide for Caregivers, Loved Ones, and People with a AIDS [1994]*
- *Elder Care Activities: 105 Great Activities You Can Do at Home, in Assisted Living, a Retirement Community, or in a Nursing Home [2013]*
- *Perspectives on Care at Home for Older People [2013]*
- *Conscious Acts of Grace—Gifts of Love and Kindness at the End of Life [2010]*
- *Knocking on Heaven's Door: the Path to a Better Way of Death [2013]*
- *The Preemie Parents' Companion: the Essential Guide to Caring for Your Premature Baby in the Hospital, at Home, and Through the First Years [2000]*
- *Spiritual Midwifery [2002]*
- *Keeley Meditation: Free Your Mind [2012]*
- *The Complete Guide to Medicaid Nursing Home Costs: How to Keep Your Family Assets Protected—up to Date Medicaid… [2008]*
- *Comrades in Health: U.S. Health Internationalists, Abroad and at Home [2013]*
- *Caregiver Relief: A Stress Management Guide [2013]*
- *Seniors at Large [2012]*
- *Cancer Caregiving A-to-Z: An At-home Guide for Patients and Families [2008]*
- *Conversations at the Nursing Home: A Mother, a Daughter, and Alzheimer's [2013]*
- *Massachusetts General Hospital Handbook of General Hospital Psychiatry [2010]*

- *Angels at the Door [2014]*
- *Caregiving Tips A-Z [2008]*
- *Making Myself at Home in a Nursing Home [2012]*
- *Supporting People with Dementia at Home: Challenges and Opportunities for the 21st Century [2012]*
- *Jekel's Epidemiology, Biostatistics and Preventive Medicine [2013]*
- *A New Look at Community-Based Respite Programs: Utilization, Satisfaction, and Development [2014]*
- *Waiting at the Gate: Creativity and Hope in the Nursing Home [2014]*
- *How to Find Someone to Care for Your Aging Person at Home [2010]*
- *Providing Good Care at Night for Older People: Practical Approaches for Use in Nursing and Care Homes [2011]*

**Some of these books would be logical sources for more detailed information on topics that will be just touched on here.** There were 40 results for the Amazon Kindle ebooks. Expanding the search to all books on amazon.com with the same "nursing care at home" topic gave 291 items. You will not suffer from a shortage of reading matter, if you wish.

**From the 40 titles listed above, we can make some distinctions about what our book does and does not cover: we cover nursing care for the chronically ill at home, including the elderly,** but

- not premature babies,
- not end-of-life, hospice care,
- not respite care for caregivers, and…unsurprisingly…
- not nursing wild birds.

Those who want to explore topics not covered here are directed to some of the titles listed above, or the titles that come from a search that includes both printed and ebooks.

**Subsequently, we became aware of an exceptionally complete treatise on home care,** Tena L. Scallan's excellent *The Ultimate Compassionate Guide to Caregiving: A Simple Blueprint for Dealing with Today's Healthcare Crisis Combined with Years of Wisdom and Sound Advice,* published in 2015 and available in paperback and ebook formats from Amazon, a book which gives finely detailed advice on the non-medical care of patients in the home, advice which we summarize in our appendix, "Custodial Care at Home," a book we urge our readers to obtain to supplement our own, which has more of a medical management emphasis. Similarly, in 2015 was published *The Successful Caregiver's Guide*, by Rick Lauber (2015), particularly valuable for those who have to move their loved ones to a care facility. A third fine resource, also published in 2015, is Dr. Nanette J. Davis's *The ABCs of Caregiving, Part 2.* (Davis, 2015)

We have organized the first part of our book along the lines of the traditional questions a journalist would ask, though in a somewhat different order: Who? What? When? Where? Why? How?

We will start with **why.** As Stephen R. Covey advised in his *The 7 Habits of Highly Effective People*, one should "start with the end in mind."

# CHAPTER 1

# WHY HOME, NOT A NURSING HOME, OR HOSPICE?

**Why would your patient rather be at home?** The people, places, and things are familiar. It's comfortable. **Why do you want to care for the patient at home?** You want to be together. You distrust care given by others, especially at a distance. In some cases, home care is less expensive.

**In a nursing home,** there is a community of patients, some whom your patient would like and some less attractive. There are schedules with limited flexibility and personnel with limited time to provide care. The nursing home is generally at a significant distance from the patient's friends and family, inhibiting visiting and monitoring the care, as will the rules of the facility. Physicians may visit, reducing the need to travel, a plus.

**In a hospice,** it is acknowledged that the illness is terminal, and the goal is patient comfort, an advantage. However, some families and some patients may well not want to accept this prognosis, and there is always a concern that being labeled as "terminal" may lead to receiving poorer care.

**Home care** can be a blessing. As written about my [DWC's] wife's situation seven years after choosing to be home rather than in a hospice (Cooper, 2011):

*"…Tina was very fragile when she first came home. Her needs were many—ventilator-dependent, unable to speak, tube-fed, unable to eat or drink by mouth; physical therapy to keep her joints pliable, causing pain no matter how gently it was done, and medication being given on schedule day and night, interrupting the little sleep she was able to find amidst all the new noises and activity in her room.*

*While her body remained fragile, Tina's spirit grew strong. (Her complaining consisted of a frown on her face.) She withstood the changes in her health condition with the attention she received from the nurses, each one caring for her as a friend as well as a patient."* [Terry Bush, LPN.]

*She's been home for seven years since then. Through my IBM retirees' medical benefits, we have had round-the-clock nursing, first through an agency and then from nurses we have obtained on our own. Most of our nurses have been with us for years, as Tina is a cooperative and cheerful patient, always appreciative of the care she receives. Here, "TLC" is "Tina-Loving Care." There have been some scary times, including several bouts of pneumonia, and many trips to the doctor in our special van. There have also been lovely times. We say "every day is a blessing." Every day is Valentine's Day….*

*Tina still cares about her friends, her family, her nurses, keeps up with the news, and relishes the documentary and music channels on TV. She chats on the phone, spends an hour or two out of bed in her wheelchair daily, and provides an inspiration to those who know her. She is our heroine.*

Now, 2016, five years after that was written, Tina's condition is somewhat worse, with significant losses in cognition and ability to communicate, but she still usually indicates she enjoys her life, and we are still happy that she continues to be with us.

# CHAPTER 2

# WHERE? ORGANIZING YOUR HOME

**Home care brings major changes to the home.** The patient may need the largest of your bedrooms…to fit a hospital bed, monitoring and life-support equipment, space to maneuver a Hoyer lift, storage for clothing and frequently used medical supplies. Because of the frequent interruptions occasioned by treatments, medications, and feedings, a Significant Other will likely find it advantageous to sleep elsewhere in the home. A television, a CD player, and a radio and a reading lamp help in providing entertainment for the bedridden patient. We subscribed to a wide spectrum of cable TV channels and Netflix, though only a few became favorites. And over the years, an abundance of DVDs have been added to the library. (Cooper, 2011)

**You'll need a surprising amount of room** to store your wheelchair, lift, disposable absorbent materials (disposable underwear), pads, gloves, equipment tubing and associated filters and connectors, your oxygen supplies (tanks, concentrator), medical record files, feeding supplies, *etc.*

**Preparation of medications and feeding materials** normally occurs in a kitchen setting, but **you need to set aside an area**

separate from what the family uses for preparing and eating meals. If the patient cannot safely swallow, you will need to post signs that say, "Nothing to swallow, NPO" [NPO is *nil per os*, Latin for "nothing by mouth].

**We found it beneficial having a spare bedroom** for the nurses to use when scheduling or weather complications made their coming and going more difficult. **You may need to remove some rugs for safety and even an occasional door** if there is difficulty getting a wheelchair or stretcher through it. We were glad to have a laundry room right by the bedroom. **We added a ramp to access the front door** and were fortunate to have the bedrooms on the ground floor. **Consideration must be given to how the patient will be evacuated in case of fire, and we prohibited any flames anywhere in the home. Fire alarms were installed in several rooms and front and back door areas had fire extinguishers.**

**In case of emergency, one wants help to have easy access, so we did not lock our doors. For an alarm and somewhat for our protection, we had a dog,** one who raised a fuss when strangers came, although no one was ever bitten. The nurses came to like having Brandy (and later, Colette), especially the nurses who handled the overnight shifts.

Having retired somewhat sooner than expected, I (DWC) was able to be at home generally 20 hours a day, to provide some help, monitor activities, handle paperwork, and occasionally socialize with our two patients. **Visitors were rare, as we did not invite many in, partly to limit risk of infection and partly due to the loss of friends and family after we moved to the country.**

# CHAPTER 3

# WHAT? EQUIPMENT AND SUPPLIES

**You will probably be surprised how much "stuff" is involved in providing skilled nursing care at home.** The particulars will depend on your patient's condition. Here, we look at the situation for our quadriplegic, ventilator-dependent, tube-fed patient.

## EQUIPMENT

**The material in italics here comes from *Ting and I* (Cooper, 2011); the non-italicized portions have been added subsequently.**

### Computer

*Our computer and computer skills aided us greatly once we replaced the nursing agency.*

*We pay the nurses on Thursday or on their last shift of the week. The spreadsheet program on our computer enables us to print out the details of date, shift, hours worked, gross pay, deductions (FICA and Medicare), and net pay. Two copies are made, one for the nurse, the other for her to sign and return to us for our records.*

*The insurers want similar information, monthly. The federal government also wants much the same information monthly, along with the deductions and the matching employer "contributions" to FICA and Medicare.*

*Quarterly and annual reports for the state and federal government are required as well. I do the first draft. We have an accountant to prepare the final draft. The same happens with the preparation of the IRS W-2 income tax forms at the end of the year.*

*Fun!*

**"Leveraging the Power of Technology to Help with Caregiver Duties" is the title of an excellent blog article** contributed by Nathan McVeigh (2015) to the blog lotsahelpinghands.com. Some suggestions require a computer and some do not:

1. "Access to Education and Resources"
   He contrasts illness-specific sites like cancercare.org and alz.org with more general sites like cargiveraction.org and lotsahelpinghands.com. Each has its strengths.

2. "Daily Care"
   He lists instacart.com for shopping and postmates.com for meals right away and taskrabbit.com for tasks you want to delegate.

3. "GPS Technology"
   For patients with dementia, such devices can be attached to their clothes to help find the patients. Other devices allow you to monitor patient conditions

remotely. McVeigh lists: resources.careinnovations.com/quietcare, mylively.com, lifelinesys.com/content, and life360.com.

4. "Personal Emergency Response Systems"
   Examples given are medicalert.com and lifealert.com.

5. "Medication Reminders"
   A full-service pharmacy is pillpack.com. Reminder services include tabsafe.com and medminder.com, and there are phone aps.

6. "Wireless Home Monitoring"
   These are advertised on TV and can alert you to a fall or an unauthorized departure.

7. "Software Applications and Health Tracking Tools"
   Platforms such as healthvault.com and the lotsahelpinghands.com site offer storage for the multitudinous appointments often associated with caregiving.

8. "Support Communities"
   Sites such as lotsahelpinghands.com provide support for caregivers and family members. Various illnesses have their own specific support groups.

### Hospital Bed (Cooper, 2011)

*A sturdy hospital-type bed, where the upper third and the lower third can be raised or lowered electrically has proved very valuable. The full-queen bed we use is wide enough to allow easy movement of Tina onto her side and back. The width allowed me to sleep or rest beside her during the year without overnight nurses. The head rest is up for watching TV, being fed, talking on the telephone, and gastric tube and tracheostomy care. It is down for disposable diaper changes, bed baths, and shampoos.*

For our other patient, a woman in her nineties, a standard-width hospital bed was used, one roughly the width of a standard single bed. When this patient was mobile, rails had to be installed on both sides to keep her from climbing or falling out. Overnight, a belt around her waist was used for added safety, and she was connected to a bed alarm that would sound if she pulled it loose.

### Hoyer Hydraulic Lift

*Nurses tell me that back injuries are endemic to their profession. Lifting and transferring patients cause most of the injuries.*

*Tina weighs 125 pounds, rather slender at 5'5", lighter than the average adult patient. Still, the Hoyer hand-pumped hydraulic lift is a back-saver. Pump, pump, pump and up she rises, like Mary Poppins as she thinks happy thoughts. Open the faucet-like valve, and down she comes, slowly if you are careful. Tina lands onto her bed or into her wheelchair like a snowflake in the winter, a flower petal in the spring, a glider in the summer, and a leaf in the fall.*

For our elderly patient, when she was no longer able to get much value from being transferred to her wheelchair when not making a doctor visit, **we used the lift and her sling to "dangle" her above the bed,** in a posture much like sitting upright. This was believed to have cardio-vascular benefits and to keep some of her muscles in use in ways that they were not used when she was supine in bed.

### Pulse Oximeter

*Using laser light, these highly informative meters give pulse rate and the percentage oxygen saturation of the blood. Some are smaller than a deck of cards.*

*Tina's normal pulse rate is 70 to 90 per minute. Lower than that may indicate she is sleeping or may be a cause for concern. Higher than that suggests agitation or a fever.*

*Tina's normal oxygen saturation percentage ($pO_2$) is 98 to 100 percent, quite good, in response to the additional 3 liters per minute of oxygen supplied to her by the ventilator, mixed with the room air. Lower than that suggests the oxygen line has become crimped or disconnected or that there is a leak. Without the line, she registers 92–94 percent $pO_2$. Breathing room air for minutes without the ventilator, she can stay near 90 percent, the low end of the safe range, but we do not know for how long, and we are not eager to test it. In an emergency (say, a fire), she will be evacuated immediately, quite possibly without the ventilator.*

**The primary goal of the ventilator and the auxiliary oxygen supply is to keep the oxygen content of the blood high enough [above 90%] to prevent cell death.** The pulse oximeter, measuring the oxygen content at fingers or toes, where it is likely to be least, provides this vital information, along with monitoring heart rate, also vital. **It does not tell how well carbon dioxide is being removed from the blood,** so it is not the complete story on how well the respiratory equipment and the patient's respiratory system are performing.

### Ventilator

*The ventilators we have will not let Tina's respiration rate fall below 10 per minute, a value she often reaches during deep sleep. Usually, the "vent" monitors her natural breathing pattern, adding input air as she starts to breathe in, withdrawing air as she breathes out. It assists, rather than replaces, her normal respiration.*

*The ventilator is one of several pieces of equipment in Tina's room that repay some familiarity with electronics, mechanics, fluid flow and physiology, much of which I had expertise in from my career in environmental science and engineering. The ventilator displays a series of values for her breathing cycle, the most useful to us being the breath rate, f. Values of between 10 and 20 per minute are of no concern. Values in the 20s may indicate a problem. When she started to develop pneumonia, the rate went to the 30s per minute. Time to call 911.*

*The ventilator is a modern technological miracle. Sure beats an iron lung.*

Ventilator and oxygen flow settings for our two patients were somewhat different, the older patient having been diagnosed as afflicted with COPD, chronic obstructive pulmonary disorder, possibly due to smoking, which she only gave up in her forties.

### Vacuum Pump

**Respirator-dependent patients need regular clearing of the**

airways, using suction provided by a vacuum pump. A covered in-line catheter is best for this, as the covering reduces the chance of contamination on the thin tube that goes through the tracheostomy tube and into the windpipe, the trachea. Sometimes lavage is performed, introducing a few mL of saline solution into the windpipe and then rapidly removing it with the catheter. This loosens and partially dissolves mucus plugs that can block the airway. The material withdrawn is collected in a canister associated with the pump, and the canister is cleaned regularly, with soap and water and perhaps with a vinegar/water 50/50 solution used to disinfect it.

Briefly closing off the tubing coming from the pump and observing the vacuum gauge can allow one to judge whether the pump is performing properly. Sometimes weak vacuum is due to loose tubing connections, improper sealing of the top of the canister to the bottom, or excessive moisture in the filter immediately upstream from the pump, used to protect it from material or liquid escaping the canister and into the line ahead of the pump.

### Oxygen Concentrator

Tina's supplementary oxygen flow to her through her ventilator is 3 liters per minute (3 L/min). A liter is roughly a quart, and there are 28.3 liters in a cubic foot. In one day that means a volume of oxygen of

(3 L/min)(60 min/hr)(24 hr/day)= 4320 L/day

about 150 cubic feet of oxygen. To supply this with oxygen tanks would be awkward and expensive. Instead, the oxygen concentrator strips most of the nitrogen from ambient air and sends the remaining oxygen to the patient. It does so at the cost of electric power, and if the power goes out, one needs to use back-up oxygen tanks.

### Oxygen Tanks

**For traveling and for loss-of-power situations, we needed oxygen tanks.** The portable ones were filled to a pressure of about 2000 psi [pounds per square inch] and contained just under 700 liters of oxygen at room temperature and pressure [70oF, 14.7psig= 1 atm]. When used at 3L/min, these would give about 210 minutes of flow or 3.5 hours. Monitoring Tina's blood oxygen content with a pulse oximeter allowed us to lower this flow to about 1L/min for trips, without hazard.

### Electrical Generators

**We have two gasoline-powered electrical generators,** one for 5000 watts and the other for 4000 watts, our back-up to our back-up generator. They require some attention during the year, with the addition of gasoline additive to prevent fouling and with running the generators every month or two to assure they are working and to keep the gas flow lines clear. We run extension cords from the generators, and the cords have multi-outlet attachments.

**Alternatively, we could have installed a propane-powered back-up power supply system** at a cost of about $10,000, ten times what the two smaller generators cost in total. Besides the cost disadvantage, it would have been too complex for us to repair immediately if it, too, failed, and there is some concern about fire hazard in having propane in the vicinity of oxygen supplies.

### Washer–Dryer

*A medium or large wash is done each of our four shifts each day. Pads, sheets, pillow cases, nightgowns, towels, all need washing and drying, with different frequencies.*

*When the washer needs repair? Yes, we have a backup.*

The addition of a second patient meant we ran 6 to 7 loads per day.

### Redundancy

*When possible, we have had back-ups for our equipment: two ventilators, large and small oxygen tanks to supplement the oxygen concentrator, heating and air conditioning units in Tina's room to supplement the central heating and air conditioning, a gasoline-powered 5,000-watt electrical generator to protect us from power outages, the longest of which was 95 hours. Our previous special van had two gas tanks.*

*The multitudinous disposables used daily also need to be in abundance, taking into account the possibility of delays in receiving shipments of them. We have a month or more of all of these, including the crucial special complete nutrition liquid. This much stuff required a room for storage, our dining room, and a sharp, detail-oriented home manager, Barbara George, to track them.*

Note that I soon bought a second, back-up gasoline-powered generator once our elderly patient became ventilator-dependent.

## MEDICATIONS AND NUTRITION

*By our seventh year of home care, we were using the gastric tube to administer the following medications, vitamins, and foods the indicated number of times per day: morphine sulfate\* (eight), Carafate (sucralfate)\* (four), Baclofen\* (three), balanced nutrition liquid\* (five), protein supplement\* (twice), Prozac\* (once), vitamins $B_6$, $B_{12}$, C\*, and MgO, K, Ca\* (each once), Fe (twice), yogurt (twice), Benadryl\* (twice), Proloprim\* (once), Ativan\* (once), cranberry juice (once), aspirin\* (once).*

*None of these was given against doctor's orders. Those with asterisks were prescribed; some were available over the counter. Keeping track of these was done by a matrix, a "chart," with rows being the items and their timing and the columns being the dates, with the intersection initialed by the nurse giving the item. Each chart noted the four chemicals to which Tina is allergic. A similar chart was developed for the many treatments needed regularly.*

*We had doctors' orders for another dozen medications on a PRN (as needed) basis. This way, we were not asking the nurses to give Tina something not medically authorized.*

*In feeding, there are two easy ways to go wrong: too much food or too little. For Tina, we started with five cans of a 250-calorie balanced-nutrition drink. With the yogurt and juice, the total was nearly 1,400 calories. After a year or so, my 125-pound love had gained definite chub. Creases had formed in the skin* on her back, and they were getting irritated. We cut back by one can a day to four per day, about 1,200 calories in all. Two feedings with whole cans were replaced by two feedings with half cans plus water. Slowly, the former sylph returned. At roughly 4,000 calories per pound of weight gained or lost, losing ten pounds should have taken about

$$(10 \text{ lb}) \times (4,000 \text{ cal/lb}) / (250 \text{ cal/day}) = 160 \text{ days},$$

probably not too different from what transpired. Physicists love equations.

My mother represented the other way to go wrong. She ate like a bird, a fussy bird, at that. In three months she went from about 125 pounds to about 110, a loss of 5 pounds per month. A similar estimate indicated she was getting $5 \times 4,000 / 30 = 700$ too few calories a day. I summarized this for her: "Eat or die!" She started eating more. "Eat and live!" became the rallying cry.

Yes, we know that a more accurate value for calories to poundage is 3600 calories per pound. There are subtle effects of metabolism that make even this number an approximation. Still, caloric intake and patient activity determine weight gain or loss.

## Prescriptions: Liquids Cost Us Much More Than Pills

**In three cases we found that getting the same amount of active medicine in liquid form was much more expensive than getting it in pill form.**

**One patient needed morphine for pain.** The liquid form (a solution) cost us about $2000 per year. The same dosing, obtained by crushing a tablet and dissolving it in water, cost about $1000 per year. This was the cost of our co-pay; the insurer paid much more.

**The simple salt compound KCl, potassium chloride,** cost us about $200 per year as pills and cost our insurer about $1000 per year. The same dosage in liquid form cost about three times as much. Again, the pill could be crushed and dissolved in water; we did.

**The third example was the medication that is available over-the counter as Pepcid and as a prescription as famotidine.** The monthly dose of the liquid version of the prescription had a "usual and customary" cost of $530, of which we would pay $45, and the insurer and drugstore would pay the rest. A month of the prescription pills had a cost of $30 of which we would pay $6. A month of the over-the-counter Pepcid pills would cost us $20, and would not be covered by insurance. **Note the much higher cost of the liquid form,** which is easily obtained at home by dissolving two pills in a few ounces of water.

### Side Effects

*Powerful medications rarely have only one effect on the body. The other effects, "side effects," one hopes will be benign or mild. We have to be watchful for them, especially during the early applications of a given medicine.*

*Tina is allergic to a few meds, and these are prominently listed at the top of each medication scheduling chart. If a new drug being started is related to any of these, we watch with particular care.*

From the various nursing and medical handbooks, one can read a listing of typical, unusual, and rare side effects, with some highlighted as serious. In home care, the prescribing physicians are relying on nurses and family to detect such adverse reactions.

Less obvious is the interaction of two or more drugs to aggravate the side effects of each. We noticed Tina was losing her hair, which would have been very upsetting for her. We spotted two of her drugs that had this as a rare side effect. Combined, apparently, they were more of a problem. Checking with the doctor, we dropped or found a substitute for one of the drugs, and this problem went away. Surprisingly, one or more of her medications has led to a lovely waviness of her hair.

Drug interactions are hard to detect and probably more common than most people think. The number of combinations goes up rapidly with the number of drugs. For drug A and drug B, there is only 1 combination, AB. For A and B and C, there are 3 combinations: AB, AC, BC. For A and B and C and D, there are AB, AC, AD, BC, BD, CD, six paired combinations. For N drugs, each new drug adds (N-1) more pairs. Note, too, that three or more drugs lead to sets of triadic combinations: A and B and C and D have: ABC, ABD, ACD, and BCD. No wonder surprises turn up! We traced Tina's only seizure episode to such a three-drug combination.

Did I mention that physicists love equations?

# SUPPLIES

**A surprising amount of material is needed to care for a bedridden patient.**

For a patient getting a **disposable diaper change every four hours**, you need 6x30=**180 diapers per month**. We bought them in cases of 60, and we averaged four cases per month per patient, as there were times when the diapers needed changing more often.

We found that using a liner along with the disposable diaper prevented leakage, and we used about **1 case of 200 liners per month**.

Activities involving contacting the patient were carried out with gloved hands for the mutual protection of patient and caregiver. We used about **1500 gloves per patient per month,** 50 per day. Gloves came in packages of 1000.

Disposable wipes were consumed at the rate of approximately 2 cases of about 500 **pre-wetted wipes per month, 1000 per month,** 33 per day.

A patient fed through a gastric tube needs a supply of paren-teral complete-nutrition feeding fluid. **One of our patients took about 1200 calories of this daily, and the other took about 1000 calories of much the same liquid daily. The latter received supplementary cranberry juice and liquid yogurt, bringing her to near 1200 calories a day,** as well; she had shown weight gain over period of months when she had been given 250 more calories per day. Excess weight is a problem for the patient, especially for the skin over bony areas, and for the caregivers, who need to roll and transfer the patient frequently.

**Cleaning supplies are consumed in prodigious amounts.** We also ran the washer-drier combination every shift, thus three or four times a day, even with one patient. Adding a second patient led to washes 6 to 7 times per day.

**Ventilator supplies ordered per patient monthly included:**

- Disposable inner cannula (30/month)
- In-line suction catheter (15/month)
- Ventilator circuit tubing (2/month)
- 50' oxygen line (2/month)
- Circuit filter (2/month)
- Ventilator filter (2/month)
- Flexible connector for trach site (15/month)
- Tracheotomy ties (20/month)
- Suction tubing (4/month)
- Heat and moisture economizers (HMEs, 30/month)
- Split gauze pads (4" x 4", 100/month)
- Cotton-tipped applicators
- Saline flushes (3mL containers)

Inventory Management

**Keeping track of supplies can be a headache. By the basic rule of organization that similar things should be kept closer together than dissimilar things,** one can put the material where shortages and excesses become evident. We ordered supplies by using a computer spreadsheet to help predict needs and record ordering and acquisition.

For each supplier we made a monthly order (at staggered dates during the month), going down the list of items they supplied, generally re-ordering what we had ordered the month before.

A better system of inventory management would be to set up the following tabulation on a spreadsheet:

| ITEM, UNITS | AVG USE PER MONTH | NOW (DATE) ON HAND | IN STOCK # MONTHS |
|---|---|---|---|
| Diapers, case (4x15) | 4 | 3 | 0.75 |
| Gloves, box (1000) | 1.5 | 2 | 1.3 |
| Wipers, case (500) | 2 | 2 | 1.0 |

The variability of arrivals of supplies suggests one should aim to have at least half-a-month's worth on hand.

## Redundancy of Suppliers

Where feasible, it is prudent to have more than one supplier. Fortunately, some of the material we used was also obtainable from the local supermarket in roughly equivalent products.

# CHAPTER 4

# WHEN? STARTING, SCHEDULING, STOPPING

**"On your mark, get set, go!"** It's easier to win the race if you have a head start, so get started early on: **where, who, how** care will be given later.

**The hospital will likely give you a specialist to aid in the transition to home, but you will quickly be on your own unless you hire a nursing agency,** which would simplify your tasks but at higher costs and give you less control than you would have if you were managing the care yourself. We started with an agency, learned from them, saw how to do better, and started hiring our own nurses. Without an agency, you'd quickly have to advertise for, interview, and orient your new nurses, and you might not have your systems in place to demonstrate the requirements of the job.

**Advertise** in local publications and on the Internet.

**Ask** people who might have employed nurses before.

**Interview** in the home: name, address, training, experience, availability, references, extra capabilities. Would they fear or be allergic to your pet? Rule out smoking on the job. In case of emergency, can they help evacuate the patient? Do they have any physical disabilities that would keep them from moving the patient in bed and transferring the patient to and from the bed? **Keep your questions task-related. Do not ask questions that might suggest you would discriminate unfairly or illegally.** As you converse, try to determine whether they are sufficiently intelligent and articulate and pleasant to make you comfortable having them in your home. After they leave, write your comments on your home-made form, so you don't forget, and give them a tentative grade (A down to F). **Don't write down something that might embarrass you later, if it came to light.**

**Call references,** unless you have ruled the candidate out. If a majority of the references for a candidate don't respond or are lukewarm, rule that nurse out. You are looking for "wonderful," "great," "outstanding," *etc.* from people she/he worked for. Ask how long they were employed, doing what, and would the employer hire the person again. Again, do not ask questions that might suggest you would discriminate unfairly or illegally. Friends of the candidate can be expected to be enthusiastic. **Consider using a detective agency to do a background check.**

**Ask what nursing credential the candidate has, RN or LPN.** Registered Nurses (RNs) have more training than Licensed Practical Nurses (LPNs), and they typically get about 50% more per hour. An LPN with many years of experience is probably equivalent to a new RN, although the latter will have more "book learning." **We had a mix, but paid all the same (to forestall rivalry or jealousy), attracting LPNs from much farther away than RNs.**

In the rest of this chapter, and in the Exhibits, which are in the back of the book, we will show the different forms, the "charts," we created for scheduling shifts, treatments, medications, assessments, *etc.*

# SHIFT SCHEDULE, EXHIBIT #1

**First is an example, Exhibit #1, of the schedule we posted for our nurses, usually at least a month in advance.** The shifts varied in starting and ending times to accommodate certain nurses. The initials identified the nurses, whose names are not given in the sample.

**This schedule's title indicates the schedule was posted over a month in advance and was considered tentative, but probable.** The August schedule was posted May 31. The first column is the work date. Next is the first shift, usually 8 a.m. to 4 p.m., followed by an afternoon-evening shift (e.g., 4 p.m. to 10 p.m.) and an overnight shift (usually 10 p.m. to 8 a.m.). We did not give the overnight nurses an overnight pay-rate differential, but the longer hours and the relative lack of activity on the overnight shift made it adequately attractive to keep it staffed.

**If a nurse worked a shift routinely for a prolonged period, she essentially "owned" it,** so she could plan her life outside the job easily. If she could not work a shift, she had to get a substitute from the staff of about ten nurses. They could exchange hours or money or both, and they did so freely and reliably. Once in agreement, they would cross out the initials originally on the schedule and replace them with their own. **We paid the nurses before they actually worked for the coming week,** so they had to work out their settlement with each other if they made it after we made the payroll. In one or two instances, we lost money due to a nurse's failure to work the pre-paid shifts. One such loss was about $1400, however, from a nurse we had fired after pre-paying her but allowed to finish her week; she failed to show up.

**Soon after arriving, the oncoming nurse would discuss with the nurse being relieved what significant activities had occurred.** She would also read the communications book and then look at the comprehensive charting book.

## COMMUNICATIONS BOOK

**Bound composition notebooks were used and eventually stored when full.** Notifications of the nurses, requests for supplies or substitutes, comments on nursing practice were entered by management and staff at will. This did not replace the more formal nursing assessment forms, however.

## CHART BOOK

As much as physicists like equations, **nurses dislike documentation.** It is often a thorn in their side and frequently perceived as time taken away from the actual job of "nursing," giving care to the patient. But it is also recognized as required by law and necessary for optimal care. Nursing combines giving care with making assessments and recording both.

**We have, over many years, developed our home-care documentation to be user-friendly and require minimal charting time, thus decreasing time taken away from caring for the patient.** Some documents have taken the form of checklists requiring only initialing the completed actions for medication administration and treatments. Our assessment sheet, which is organized by systems and is a one-page, two-sided document, provides for merely checking-off or circling most assessment criteria. Minimal writing is necessary—but space is also available when needed.

**Our forms have worked well in our practice.** Whether used for nursing professionals or family in-home caregivers, these are merely "to-do" lists and "observation" forms. **They provide a list of what needs to be done and when it must be done.** Additionally, by noting what, when, or how something looked today, for example, it provides a means for comparison to see if there is improvement or a decline from one day to another. Once written and/or checked off, it no longer has to be remembered. It can be factually referenced later, if needed. It eliminates "I think...." And if the area, box, or section of the form isn't completed, it's a reminder that something wasn't done and needs to be. In the nursing profession there is an adage: "if it wasn't charted, it wasn't done. "

**In this part of the book, we give a brief description of the documents we use, leaving more detailed descriptions to the appended material near the end of the book. Please refer to the Exhibits section for document samples.** Some information has been changed for patient privacy or redacted for space limitations. Field descriptions and medical information pertaining to the forms appear also.

## PHYSICIAN'S ORDERS: DAILY AND PRN MEDICATIONS, EXHIBIT #2A, EQUIPMENT & TREATMENTS, EXHIBIT #2B

**We obtain renewed medication and treatment orders from the patient's primary care physician every 90 days.** This is done for insurance purposes as well as to provide the nurses with ongoing orders for their practice. Generally, it is nothing more than a list of all that is necessary for the patient's continuing care. Once submitted to the physician, he evaluates and signs off on the orders, and they are returned to us. See the Exhibits section of this book for details.

## EMERGENCY PLAN, EXHIBIT #3

**This needs to be near the front of the patient's "chart," or book, although unlikely to be needed.**

Responses for potential emergencies are described for the following:

- Loss of electrical power
- Loss of ventilator
- Fire
- Choking

Not all possible emergencies can or should be covered, just those whose severity and probability are greatest.

## REFERENCE INFORMATION AND CONTACTS, EXHIBIT #4

This merely provides a complete and detailed listing of patient specifics, physician contacts, and other pertinent information pertaining to the household and the patient.

- Patient information
- Miscellaneous contact information
- Physician and pharmacy information

- Emergency transport information
- Vent settings

Please refer to the Exhibits section for this document sample.

# MONTHLY NURSING TREATMENT FORMS: EXHIBIT #5A (PAGE 1) & EXHIBIT #5B (PAGE 3)

**Simply stated, this document is a "to-do" list of requirements for the patient's care. Like any "to-do" list, the purpose is to ensure what needs to be done is not forgotten.** It eliminates forgetting to perform tasks and prevents essential information from being omitted during the nurses' reporting-off period. In addition, it provides a method to track and reorder inventory, since it provides what equipment is used and how often it must be replaced. Lastly, besides assuring that essential activities are completed, it holds nurses or caregivers responsible for ensuring the item was done, as well as done correctly.

These tasks are done periodically, such as on each shift or on a daily, weekly or monthly basis. They include patient treatments, such as dressing changes, as well as changing equipment to ensure continued and optimal operation…for example, changing the in-line suction apparatus. In our practice, we also use the Treatment Sheets as reminders to the nursing staff to, for example, check the Communication Book, and we try to ensure their practice is safe for them by reminding them to use Universal Precautions.

**Toward the back of this book, two exhibits of this patient's six-page document are provided to illustrate various time frames and how to depict when a certain task may require attention when not completed on a daily basis.**

# DAILY MEDICATION ADMINISTRATION RECORD—PAGE 1: EXHIBIT #6A
# PRN MEDICATION ADMINISTRATION RECORD—PAGE 6: EXHIBIT #6B

**Often referred to as the "MAR," this follows the same pattern as the treatment form.** However, instead of the activities which need to be performed, the administration of medications and feedings are noted.

**This is another "to-do" list but is solely dedicated to the administration and application of medications, ointments, creams, suppositories and any other substances that may "go into or onto" a patient** for treatment of a condition prescribed by a physician. Again, only a sample of the MAR is provided: the first and sixth pages of eight, in this patient's case, are shown.

# NURSING REVIEW/ASSESSMENT FORM: PAGE 1: EXHIBIT #7A &
# PAGE 2: EXHIBIT #7B

**Assessments are crucial for evaluating and appraising a patient.** The patient is observed in a step-by-step pattern, system-by-system. Use of touch, smell, sight, and hearing are all vital in the assessments' completion. The Assessment Form is the manner by which the assessment is documented. It provides a history of the patient's medical condition, which then allows for comparisons as well as to understand what is normal for that person.

**At the beginning of each nursing shift,** the oncoming nurse begins completion of the Nursing Review / Assessment Form. This one-page, two-sided document is used to evaluate the patient's current physical and emotional condition; log medication administrations; track treatments; ensure proper equipment settings and changes; and generally provides a permanent record to ensure vital information isn't lost or misreported. While a general physical assessment will be completed early in the shift, the form is used throughout the entire period to document any changes in the patient's condition and record completed actions.

**The form used for the patient is broken down into thirteen sections.** Most categories pertain to the major body systems. However, there are also sections for general information, equipment checks, nursing and shift identification, as well as allowing space for notes. A large amount of information is recorded simply by selecting or circling items. Not only does this serve to remind nurses what to assess and aid in its full completion, it also minimizes handwriting legibility problems.

# VENT SETTINGS

**Used for ventilator-required patients with pulmonary problems, vent settings are dictated by a pulmonologist.** For this patient, each shift, these setting are checked to ensure they are accurate and have not been mistakenly changed, which potentially could be life-threatening.

# INTAKE

**Whether the patient is able to eat by mouth or uses a gastric tube for all fluids and nutrition, the amount the patient ingests is vital to know.** Too much fluid could cause edema, hypertension (high blood pressure), and could create pulmonary problems if the fluid backs up into the lungs. Too little fluid can result is hypotension (low blood pressure) and decreased perfusion (oxygen supply) to vital organs. **Recording nutrition is imperative** to ensure that sufficient quantities of protein, water and nutrients are available to promote healing, maintain skin, and provide fuel for continued functioning of the body at the cellular level.

# NEUROLOGIC

**The neurologic system is comprised of the brain, brain stem, spinal cord, which completes the central nervous system, and also included are various nerves located throughout the entire body, the peripheral nervous system.** It is a complex system, using neurochemicals and transmitters and cellular structures to take external input from the environment via our senses and internal input from bodily functioning to transform them into usable, functional, and creative data which we perceive as life.

This section is used to assess and detail neurologic function and changes throughout the shift. In general, only two main points are assessed for this patient.

# RESPIRATORY

**The respiratory system ensures the body is provided with oxygenated blood** via the smallest functioning unit in the lungs, the alveolus. It is at this cellular level that **carbon dioxide is exchanged for oxygen.** In addition to the lungs, other essential members of the system include the pharynx, epiglottis, larynx, trachea, bronchus and its tapering limbs, and the associated respiratory muscles and diaphragm.

This section is used to assess and detail respiratory function and changes, throughout the shift. In addition to assessing pulmonary function and treatments, a portion reflects equipment changes that are often required on a daily basis.

# CARDIOVASCULAR

The cardiovascular system is comprised of the heart and all the blood vessels; that is, the veins and arteries. The system functions to distribute oxygenated blood received from the lungs and deliver it throughout the body via the arteries. Venous return to the heart via veins takes deoxygenated carbon-dioxide-rich blood back to the heart to return it to the lungs for oxygenation and CO2 removal. Assessment of this system includes blood pressure readings and heart rate, which are detailed under Vital Signs (V/S), as well as pulses, tissue perfusion and fluid backup called "edema". This section is used to assess and detail cardiac and venous function and changes throughout the shift.

# GASTROINTESTINAL

The gastrointestinal system, often abbreviated as "GI" system, begins at the mouth and extends throughout the body to the end of the large colon at the anus. It processes food using many complex sequences and functions to transform bulk into minute substances for use at the cellular level. While processing food, the system also conserves water and returns it to the body, and prepares what is unusable for elimination via stool. The GI system is comprised of the oral cavity, esophagus, stomach, small intestine, and large intestine. However, various other organs also contribute and play key roles in the proper functioning of this system. These accessory organs are the salivary glands, gallbladder, pancreas, and liver.

**Patients that do not obtain nutrition by mouth require all substances for survival be directly received into the stomach or the jejunum section of the small intestine via a tube placed surgically. This patient had a percutaneous endoscopic gastrostomy (PEG) to place a tube into the stomach, out from stomach wall through the skin to outside the body with which to deliver nutrition.** Daily care and assessment is essential for the continued functioning of the tube, and this section is used to assess and detail gastrointestinal changes throughout the shift.

# GENITOURINARY

**The urinary system captures liquid waste from the body and voids it by way of urine production and elimination.** Through a process initiating from the kidneys, which are located on each flank or side of the body, all fluid is filtered. What is necessary for the body at that time is restored: non-essential substances as well as extra fluid are eliminated. Other organs involved in the voiding process include the ureters which bring urine to the bladder where it is stored and eventually eliminated by way of the urethra.

**The reproductive system is close to the urinary system, although these are two separate systems. Both systems are assessed at the same time**, and although no separate fields are dedicated to the genital-reproductive system, and since menses has stopped, it is documented as one system for this patient.

**For this patient, urinary catheterization is not performed. The**

patient has routine Undergarment (disposable diaper) changes at regular three-to-four-hour intervals with implementation of absorbent inserts to help keep skin dry. Another option is urinary catheterization, which allows for urine to flow freely: a tube is inserted into the urethra until reaching the bladder. Urine then flows into and is collected in a bag for accurate measurement and assessment. Catheterization can be done intermittently throughout the day without leaving a tube in place. Sterile procedure must be followed to keep from causing an infection in the urinary tract.

## MUSCULOSKELETAL / SKIN

Also essential to the body are the muscles and skin. Muscles provide metabolism, strength, and functionality for motor actions or even tasks related to the most basic functions such as breathing and pumping of the heart. Skin is the largest system of the body. It acts as a protective layer, promotes temperature regulation by perspiration, and is an indicator of other bodily system functionality, such as cardiovascular, respiratory, and gastrointestinal intake and elimination.

Skin breakdown can cause severe and devastating effects. Skin breakdown starts as a non-blanchable area (one that doesn't turn pink from white when pressure is removed from the site), a reddened patch often on a bony prominence. Tissue breakdown occurs quickly, and in the most severe cases, can extend to the bone. Depending on the patient's underlying condition, breakdown can occur in as little as two hours. Once breakdown starts, it is difficult to stop and recover from the process.

This section is used to assess and care for the muscles, bones, and skin as well as document care to eliminate skin breakdown throughout the shift.

## PSYCHO-SOCIAL

**Psycho-social aspects of a patient pertain to the emotional, psychological, and social characteristics.** They are assessed and documented to provide insight on how well the patient is adapting to the illness and the care and how they outwardly present concerns or emotional well-being.

This section is used to assess and detail psycho-social well-being and changes throughout the shift.

## BOWEL ELIMINATION / CHANGE RECORD: EXHIBIT #8

Another form we developed was to solely track fecal output. **One of the most challenging aspects in nursing is bowel regulation, especially in a bed-ridden patient on liquid nutrition.** Optimal bowel function requires bulk, as in fresh vegetables, fruit, and whole grains. Hydration is vital so that the body doesn't take all the fluid from the stool, resulting in an impaction. However, too much hydration may result in fluid overload, affecting electrolyte imbalances, edema, and backup in the cardiac and pulmonary systems. Bowel function also requires movement, both by the body and by peristaltic activity of the gastric and colon muscles. **Medications can also impair normal function, producing either too much output or not enough. For example, opioid pain medications can induce constipation.**

**To track, record, and provide ease in reporting, we developed the Bowel Elimination / Undergarment Change Record.**

At one glance, any nurse or caregiver can look to see a past and present status of bowel elimination, including quantity and quality of the stool—both very important. It also provides a time when disposable undergarments (often referred to as "adult diapers") changes are to be made. So it performs a dual task: when to do a change (for us, usually q3h=every 3 hours)—and what occurred during each change.

To ensure elimination, we have in place measures to promote bowel activity because we were able to provide the physician with documentation. Physician-ordered bowel protocols include daily administration of Miralax, alternate days of other bowel-movement promoting medications, and PRN medications to help evacuation if necessary after 48 hours without such movements. As such, bowel elimination is no longer the problem it once was, and it hasn't been a significant problem for quite some time.

**There is another purpose of the Bowel Elimination / Undergarment Change Record besides keeping track of bowel function. It provides a means to decrease the risks of bedsores.** Once a bedsore begins, usually as a benign, small reddened area that doesn't turn white when the skin is depressed (non-blanchable), it can quickly turn into an open wound that can damage skin, fat tissue, and muscles, continuing to the bone. By changing these disposable undergarments often, we get to assess any breakdown at a very early stage. Since the patient is being moved, this activity allows for improving general skin care with treatments such as applying lotions to the back, and for auscultating lung sounds with a stethoscope, or performing pulmonary treatments.

Wetness and pressure are two contributors to bedsores that are also decreased by using frequent undergarment changes. Urine and feces are caustic to skin during prolonged exposure. Changing undergarments at regular intervals reduces the time the patient's skin is in contact with these. After cleaning and drying the skin, we apply a water-proof ointment, such as A+D, to the skin as further protection, providing a barrier from these corrosive, acidic substances.

Constant pressure on the skin at bony prominences, such as the coccyx bone at the base of the spine, is also reduced during the disposable diaper changes, as the patient must be rolled to do the change. Even limited changing of positions throughout the course of the day greatly enhances the viability of the skin. It relieves pressure from lying on the bones, decreases shearing forces that occur as the body moves downward in bed by gravity, and provides enhancement to blood flow. This does not replace turning and positioning a regular intervals; it just adds a beneficial factor.

This two-sided form is merely a table. Completion requires only the nurse's initials and use of a code to quantify and qualify the stool.

## RX MEDICATION TRANSLATION: EXHIBIT #9

The generic and brand names of the medications are listed here, both in brand name order and in generic name order.

## STOPPING...PULLING THE PLUG

Both of our patients at home expressed the desire to continue

**to live, even with restrictions, and neither had "Living Wills" or Do Not Resuscitate (DNR) orders, which indicate the situations under which they would not want heroic efforts undertaken to save their lives.** This made our decisions easy in case something life-threatening should occur. The younger patient has had over a decade of life that she has generally enjoyed after her life-threatening episode in the hospital. The elderly patient, after nearly dying in the hospital, returned home, had a few "good" months, then lapsed into a period of long sleeps and only occasional lucidity, sometimes seeming to enjoy the company of her nurses and relatives, but usually seeming to be unaware.

Based on my experience with my wife, I [DWC] wrote the following several years ago:

*Some people argue that it is a waste to spend our resources on the disabled, especially as they get older. I disagree.*

*We value things on the basis of their usefulness and their scarcity. Water is useful, but widely available, thus generally inexpensive. Silver has practical and monetary uses and is relatively scarce, so it is much more expensive than water.*

*We do not know how long we will live. As we get older, we know there is less time left; it is scarcer. If we can make good use of it, enjoy it, be helpful, whatever, then the scarcity enhances its value. Even if what we do is not as good as it was years before, the years we have left can be quite precious. Tina's life is precious, as is my own.*

*Some social planners come from another perspective, viewing* public funds for medical care as investments. Babies who are unwanted or unlikely to survive do not merit investment, in this view. Your productive value goes up as you grow up, become educated, enter the work force. Toward retirement, your productivity may decline. At the very least, you have only a few more years in which to produce. These planners are reluctant to "invest" much more in you. Time to "pull the plug" on Grandpa or Grandma. Get that Do Not Resuscitate (DNR) order signed and let them expire with the next heart attack. This approach is "rational" from a public-expenditure viewpoint, though it takes no account of the value of the ill person to himself and those who care about him. It is part of a slippery slope that goes from not treating to euthanizing.

Tina's care has been expensive. We've spent money and IBM has spent more and Medicare has had a share. We certainly expected to help pay our medical costs. IBM recruited me partly though the attractiveness of its medical benefits program, which I knew we might someday need. When IBM wanted to cut its work-force, I volunteered, again considering future medical coverage needs. That leaves Medicare: decades of withdrawals from my pay checks have gone to this program, with the notional "locked-box account" for coverage of my family and me. As with other insurance, some people end up needing more and others less, a lottery of sorts. Fair enough, we thought. Now, some suggest we are "selfish" to be getting "more than our share" of medical coverage. We are not exactly winners of a lottery, but no one argues that winners of lotteries are "selfish" for collecting "more than their share."

Although I am glad we have done what we could for my [DWC's] mother, it is less clear that she benefited from the heroic efforts made in her final year.

## MOVING ON

**Sometimes, stopping will be less dire: the patient is cured, or the patient is not cured but needs a different environment to heal.**

# CHAPTER 5

# WHO? HIRING AND MANAGING NURSES

**Having had some shifts that were not covered and some nurses that were sub-par while we were using a local agency to provide nurses**, we decided to hire our own, advertising in local newspaper classified sections, interviewing, and orienting them to our procedures once hired. Our experiences as related in *Ting and I* are in italics, followed by some additional material derived from subsequent years (not italicized).

## MANAGING NURSES (COOPER, 2011)

*Managing nurses is like trying to herd cats, I jokingly told our nurse of greatest seniority here (six years). She agreed. They are very independent. They can be warm and purr. They seem to be listening to you, and yet….*

*We have had excellent nurses, judging by their behavior and by Tina's health. I jokingly say that they are a hand-picked crew, but that the next time I have to choose, I'll use a computer. Only kidding!*

### Monitoring

*"Trust, but verify." That may seem contradictory, but both elements are needed. You cannot supervise and observe everything, and you have chosen people who are trained to do what you need and generally want to do it right. Not keeping track is a recipe for failure, however. At the least, communications have got to be confirmed as received and understood. Beyond that, good practice needs to be acknowledged and bad practice corrected. Overly close observation breeds tension and resentment, but a lack of observation may communicate that you don't care, or it simply may contribute to missing something significant.*

### Agency Woes

*We started by using a nursing agency to get our round-the-clock nursing shifts covered. The agency charged IBM about twice what it paid the nurses, which may have been a fair reflection of the need for administration and profit. The nurses they supplied were highly variable in quality, however, some excellent, some poor. Getting coverage for certain shifts, such as weekend overnights, was uncertain. Sometimes I was the overnight nurse, which I could handle as long as the night was routine, the equipment functioning properly. Sleeping or resting beside Tina, I gave medicines by the gastric tube, responded to high-pressure or low-pressure alarms from the ventilator. If we had lost electrical power, it would have been difficult though not impossible to handle alone, as I touched on above.*

## Hiring Our Own

*"Who pays the piper calls the tune." I decided to do the hiring and paying myself. The extra trouble of doing so was offset by the improvement in quality it led to. Within six months, I was hiring our own nurses, supplementing and finally replacing the agency. I advertised in the local paper, interviewed them and made the hiring decisions. We live in the country, so finding our house was part of the intelligence/diligence test. About half made it to the interview, and about half of these were hired.*

*I paid them more than the agency had paid theirs, but charged IBM less than what the agency charged, using our best approximation of the actual costs, which included a variety of government surcharges.*

*There were no "off the books" dealings, as this is a sure-fire way to get in trouble or leave you open to blackmail by a disgruntled employee. And Uncle Sam needs our money, right?*

*"You get what you pay for." I would not expect our nurses to work for nothing, and I know they don't work here only for the money. By paying wages somewhat above average and by providing a pleasant working environment, we have been able to attract and keep an outstanding crew. The doctors have commented on Tina's excellent condition and care. The nurses in the hospitals have commented on the high quality of our nurses when they have seen them in action. We have our nurses stay with Tina during her rare hospitalizations, even though we are not reimbursed for this.*

## Appreciation

While on the subject of compensation, note that showing appreciation for the help the nurses supply is important. Tina thanks her nurses for almost everything they do for her, even if they say, "You don't have to thank me." I thank them often, too, and I try to be specific when I do so.

In November, the week before Thanksgiving, we give a yearly bonus to each nurse, generally a week or two of her pay (thus 2 to 4%). The ones I am most pleased with get the upper of the bonus range.

## *Interviewing*

*Interviewing the candidates, I had to get a sense of not only their skills but also the reasons they wanted this job. The salary was attractive, especially for LPNs (Licensed Practical Nurses), who often elsewhere would get only half the hourly pay of RNs (Registered Nurses). To eliminate RN-LPN rivalry and to acknowledge that their duties at our house were identical, we paid both the same rate, giving RNs some preference in choice of shift hours.*

*Home care does not provide much career advancement, does not offer the opportunity to meet a nice, eligible doctor, does involve getting along with the family, and–in our case–a seventy-pound Golden Retriever with an alpha-dog temperament. Smoking was taboo, given the oxygen in use and the difficulty there would be in evacuating Tina safely in case of a fire. Nurses were told not to come to work with a cold, as a respiratory infection was the likeliest cause of death in cases such as Tina's.*

*The highly successful coach of Penn State's football teams, Joe Paterno, recruited far more high school quarterbacks than he was going to play in that key position. They were typically outstanding athletes, and they proved their prowess when he deployed them in other positions. When I interview, I look for something like that, some outstanding strengths that will add to our team. The nurses vary in their stronger and weaker areas, but as Rocky and Adrian said, they "fill gaps."*

## Home Atmosphere

*Some say the problem with public transportation is the public. Nurses will tell you that the problem with home care is the home. They can do their jobs under a variety of conditions, but the nature of the home can make the job pleasant or unpleasant. We tried to keep that in mind. Tina is a patient patient and a gracious and grateful one. I am appreciative, too, though businesslike in manner. I praise in public and criticize in private and try to be clear in communications. We have not only detailed shift record forms to be filled out each shift by each nurse, but also a communications notebook for information that is less technical but needs to be shared.*

*One goal is to make the job a place the staff looks forward to coming to.*

*We try to live up to our motto, "Tina comes first, but everybody counts."*

## Scheduling

*On the refrigerator in the nurses' kitchen, I post two or three* months of shift schedules. Each row is a date, and the columns are for three or four shifts, typically 4 to 10 hours each, during that date, indicating which nurse (her initials) is to be on duty. I started by giving each nurse pretty much which shifts she preferred, and then I negotiated to fill the less-popular hours. I required the nurses doing 16 hours or more a week to serve some week-end time. The 10-hour shifts were almost always overnight, from 10:00 p.m. to 8:00 a.m. If a nurse needed to take some time off, she gave up hours temporarily to another nurse or traded with other nurses. They marked up the schedule to show the revision, with my approval. If a nurse did the same shift for a month or two, she "owned" it. There was a "use it or lose it" factor. New nurses were hired to fill particular gaps, then later tended to get more hours as the occasional vacancy developed. With the help of my nursing business manager, Barbara George, we almost never had a period without nursing coverage.

## Privacy

In the home care situation, we have almost no privacy. The baby monitor connecting Tina's bedroom to the nurses' kitchen/ headquarters is almost always on. Whatever one does or says is likely to be known. The nurses, too, have little privacy, as they may readily be overheard or observed. One gets used to it, and we make some effort to back off and provide each other a bit of privacy, at times.

Of course, when you are not doing something you shouldn't, the need for privacy is less. Once or twice during the week, Tina and I lock her bedroom door, use the dimmer to turn down the lights, turn off the baby monitor, and turn on some romantic music. It's a good opportunity for each to tell the other, "I love you, every cell, every second; every molecule every moment; all ways, always."

## Why Dontcha?

"Why don't you...?" This is followed by an explanation of how you could do more, better. It's helpful, in offering an idea you may not have considered, and not helpful, in seeming to add yet another burden. My response is often along the lines of "Yes, but...."

Nurse Michele Shehata says her grandmother has a saying, "Everybody wants to fish, but no one wants to get his feet wet." When I'm given a suggestion that requires added work, I try to delegate that work to the one making the suggestion, such as the suggestion that we make "fruit and vegetable smoothies" in a blender for Tina. Delegating the suggestion to the innovator may discourage input, but it makes me feel less stressed. Often, the suggestion is not carried out, because there were good reasons why it had not been done already.

Why not make smoothies for Tina?

The benefits are small. She cannot taste the smoothie, given through a gastric tube. She is already getting a balanced nutritional diet, without evident deficiencies, although a variety of foods might provide something not known to be missing.

The problems are numerous: We keep track of everything she gets, to help interpret her responses, such as rashes, flushing, etc. We would need a standard formula for the smoothie, one that we tried out in small increments at first. The ingredients would need to be purchased, then washed and cut up and prepared in the same proportions each time. They need to be processed in the blender, with the excess saved or discarded. The blender needs to be cleaned thoroughly. Who is to be responsible for each of these steps? We have a crew of ten nurses. Which ones will do what, when? This will need to be "charted," scheduled. Right now her daily calorie intake is 1,200, and her weight seems stabilized (we almost never get her to a scale). An extra 100 calories per day would mean she might gain an extra pound each month or two, unless something else is reduced or dropped. What would we eliminate?

"Smoothies" died a natural, organic death.

### How Many Nurses?

There are 168 hours a week to be covered in round-the-clock nursing. We generally have had eight to ten nurses at one time, whose weekly hours usually ranged from about 8 to about 39, averaging roughly 16 hours per nurse. As a rule, our nurses got along very well with one another, often chatting awhile about personal matters during the change-of-shift periods, which we did not discourage. Different nurses had different strengths and weaknesses, but by the end of a week, what needed to be done got done.

### How Old?

The nurses who worked out best for us were typically forty to sixty years of age. All had been married. Almost all had children. Almost all used this as a part-time job, as we did not offer health insurance, which they typically had through other means. Compassion and intelligence were most valuable traits, and these women became the primary source of Tina's social life, as we had few friends and family who could visit us regularly. To lessen the risk of contagion, we mildly discouraged visitors.

## Male Nurse?

Only rarely has a male applied for the position. Tina would not feel comfortable with one, nor would I. We have not ended up with one.

## TLC [Tina-Loving Care]

The doctors who have treated Tina have remarked on the exceptional care she has obviously been getting. Her continued survival is little short of a miracle. We are proud of her and proud of ourselves.

# PROBLEMS

Ah, you say to yourself, perhaps, this sounds too idyllic. Were there no problems? The biggest ones were the rare but scary infections Tina contracted. She came home from the Critical Care Unit with Pseudomonas and drug-resistant methicillin-resistant Staphylococcus aureus (MRSA), common hospital-acquired infections. Her good general health and the use of antibiotics beat these back, though MRSA remains in her system. For five years there were no bedsores, a major risk in these bedridden patients, and then one developed under unusual circumstances and took many months to conquer, but we did, with added help from a wound-care specialist, Edie Fitzpatrick, RN. During the last seven years there have been a few viral respiratory infections, for which medicine can do little. Fortunately, Tina's body has fought them off. Still, each day is a minor miracle. I have encouraged the nurses who really rely on this job to get a second one, too, just in case.

Other problems? Young or inexperienced nurses generally did not do well. The 20-year-old I hired as our first overnight nurse fell asleep in her chair and remained asleep as I got up from our bed, got Tina's medications, and returned to administer them. That was grounds for termination, and I did. (Recall they once shot sentries for sleeping on duty.) During the past seven years, I fired two or three others for being asleep on the overnight shift. One of the two was in her twenties, also. Inexperienced middle-aged nurses tended to be nervous but generally worked out. There often was a willingness to learn that helped offset the lack of experience and a maturity that made them more suitable companions for Tina.

### Language Barriers

A different kind of problem arose with nurse Kim, originally from Korea. Very nice, hard-working, caring, careful. Not too good with English, unfortunately. One day she described giving medicine X when it should have been Y. No real harm done, but when she went to take another job–soon after–I was both sorry to see her go and a bit relieved. "Trust, but verify" indeed.

Even native speakers of English have some misunderstandings due to the special jargon of the nursing profession. I've kidded those trained in British schools with the witty saying that Britain and America are two countries separated by a common language.

### H1N1 Flu Shots

As mentioned above, we lost several nurses over the issue of H1N1 flu shots. One had provoked an argument prior to this that led to her dismissal, but the underlying issue seemed to be her dread of the H1N1 shot. Because the flu could be deadly to Tina, an individual nurse's desire to avoid possible side effects could not weigh heavily with us. We could not let some skip the shots while requiring the others to get them. Sorry. We lost some capable nurses.

### Ms. Take

One nurse's behavior led me to court. She was a hiring mistake, and I'll refer to her as Ms. Take. In some senses she was a hardship case. She was married, had five children and now custody of a grandchild. In her interview, Ms. Take acknowledged that she was a smoker, which was usually disqualifying. She promised never to smoke on the job, and I think she kept that promise. She was an LPN, intelligent but not well-educated, with more than a dozen years of appropriate experience. Preferring not to work overnight, she was still available for any shifts we had. That might have been a tip-off. Two of her three references did not call back, another tip-off, but the one who did was favorable toward her. Ms. Take was chubby, sloppily dressed, warm and articulate. I took a chance and hired her.

She started with a half-dozen hours per week. Eventually, she was working more than the threshold necessary to qualify for unemployment benefits. After the requisite six months of this, her performance declined. Then she missed a shift without alerting us, with an excuse that did not sound true. I warned her that she was on probation. A month and a half later, on two consecutive overnight shifts, she failed to initial the numerous boxes that document medications and feedings. I knew she was busy making beaded jewelry to sell, which was acceptable as long as she met her obligations to Tina. The morning of her second night she took home with her the shift report record, the first time anyone had ever done that. I called her, listened to her excuses, and fired her.

When the Department of Labor wanted to give Ms. Take unemployment payments because she claimed that was fired without adequate cause, I appealed. Two Administrative Trial Judge hearings, of about an hour each, followed. In the first, I presented my case, and I felt optimistic. In the second, the same judge seemed leaning toward favoring Ms. Take, who had not disputed my narrative. Subsequently, the judge found in her favor. Reasons were as follows:

–We lacked an instruction book for the nurses (though the forms made it obvious what needed to be done).
–We hadn't warned her she'd be fired if she took our property (nursing records) home (did not tell her theft was not OK?)
–You aren't supposed to be fired for a first offense, generally, and this was the first time she had failed to document medications and treatments twice in a row.

We had been warned that such judges tend to favor the employee over the employer. Looked that way. I call her Ms. Take partly because she collected a substantial amount of unemployment money and partly because she had lectured one of our staff on how to maximize child welfare payments from the state.

Because we paid well above the usual LPN wage, she could honestly maintain that she could not find a comparable job in her area. Perhaps she had outsmarted us, making herself eligible for unemployment then getting herself fired.

In two or three other cases, we succeeded in appealing unemployment compensation decisions concerning other nurses we fired for good cause.

### Live-In's Relatives

When we were still using home health aides rather than nurses, we let our foreign-born aide have her husband visit from the Mother Country for a week or two and stay with us. He was odd but not much of a problem, except that Tina thought his hands strayed once too closely to her breast. Being a slow learner, I let her twenty-something son stay for a much longer period, which came to an end when he informed me that he is "a homosexualist," not something the father of a teenage boy wants to hear, at least not this father.

### Theft

Theft occurred in the seventh year of our nursing program. A week's worth of morphine doses disappeared. A few months later, a nurse's book of Robert Frost's poetry was taken. Not long after that, cans of the protein powder supplement were taken; near Christmas, a $100 bottle of Giorgio perfume was snatched. Another book seems to be missing, and other items could well be gone without our having noticed them.

Fortunately, it is only "stuff." We alerted the nurses that they should not leave any valuables of their own behind, and we let the matter drop, but it undermined my trust in the few nurses who could not be ruled out as thieves.

**In our eleventh year, I observed a nurse leave with about $20 of cleaning supplies (gloves and wipes).** Nurses often take our large empty boxes home with them for storage use, and of course we have no objection. I saw one empty box atop a seemingly empty box by the door on my way out to walk our dog. Curious, I picked up the empty box and separated it from the box beneath, and found that the lower one was not empty, but had a box of gloves ($8) and a container of wetted wipes ($12). I realized the nurse was going to take the two boxes as though empty. Initially, I separated them, to signal that I had caught on. I quickly decided not to reveal having detected this. "Knowledge is power." Soon after, that nurse took the two boxes with her, careful not to separate them in plain view. Eventually, she will likely read this and know that I know that this attractive, intelligent, well-paid nurse took stuff from us worth a half-hour's pay. I'll give her the choice of quitting or being fired. [She quit.]

In our twelfth year, over a period of a few months, we found we were about 20 Ativan (anti-anxiety narcotic) tablets short, too many for a rare miscount or tablet drop. Since our records indicated Tina was given the tablets nightly (one per night), it meant that one of the nurses was taking the pills. We moved the pills upstairs and brought them down nightly, already dissolved in a small amount of water. An acquaintance of ours indicated the Ativan pills were in real demand. "Trust, but verify," indeed.

# EMERGENCY MANAGEMENT (COOPER, 2011)

*The first page of the three-holed binder we used for our nursing information, charts, and shift reports has had a list of instructions–and telephone numbers–to assist rapid decision-making in the event of an emergency. We have discussed a few scenarios with the staff. Rapid onset of respiratory infection and fire are the two paramount risks. We choose nurses who are strong enough and well enough to drag Tina out of our home on their own in case of a fire during the few hours a day I am typically not at home.*

*Most critical is providing two paths for air flow to Tina's lungs, so that if one is blocked, she still gets air. The tracheostomy tube that goes into her throat is curved, so that it extends downward inside the trachea (windpipe). Inside it has a small balloon, the "cuff," like a tire inner-tube, that surrounds it. This means there are two paths for air: through the tracheostomy tube in her throat or around the tube to exit normally from her windpipe to larynx, mouth, and nose. Depending on the degree of inflation of the cuff, much, little, or no air flows through the space between the cuff and the inner wall of the windpipe and on to larynx, mouth, and nose. Full inflation seals the cuff to the wall, keeping any fluids, such as saliva, from flowing into the lungs, a benefit. Full inflation prevents air from going to the vocal cords, greatly limiting the patient's ability to communicate. Full inflation means that any blockage of the trach tube cuts off air to the lungs, a dangerous condition. We use partial inflation of the cuff, giving us two ways for air to get to and from the lungs, through the trach tube or around the cuff, somewhat raising the risk of aspiration of fluid into the lungs, but lowering the risk of asphyxiation.*

We have tested our ventilators and have assured ourselves that when they are off, Tina can still inhale and exhale through them. Off, they do not assist, obviously, but they are not stopping the flow, a critical concern. They have built-in batteries, and we have back-ups for them, but if some electrical fault should cause them to stop, Tina could still breathe.

In various places around our house are stored plastic gallon jugs filled with tap water. We usually drink bottled water, as our well water is mediocre. When we lose electrical power, and even when we fire up our gasoline-powered generator, we do not have electricity for the well pump. Water for cleaning and flushing quickly becomes an issue. We once had a 95-hour (four-day) outage, when our gallon jugs were very useful.

The gallon jugs of water could be useful against a very small fire, and we have fire extinguishers in each kitchen, by each exit door.

## PAIN MANAGEMENT

Before her near-death exacerbation and aspiration pneumonia in the spring of 2004, Tina rarely complained of any pain associated with MS. This MS exacerbation that cost the remaining use of her arms and hands and nearly cost her life, also left her with painful contractures of the elbows and wrists.

The primary doctor at the hospital active in her care, Dr. Richard Walker, an internist and pulmonologist, agreed with me that we must give her protection from this pain, as it made moving her for in-bed care traumatic and threatened her will to live. The solution was morphine, and I was adamant that she be given enough, even if risky, to protect her from pain. He agreed.

*For seven years now, we have been able to shield her from that pain. In a few instances, a shortage of morphine or an oversight has left her unprotected. The resumption of that pain proved the need for the continuing pain coverage.*

*Morphine sulfate solution became harder to get in 2009. We switched to morphine sulfate pills, water soluble, thus also capable of administration through the gastric feeding tube. We hadn't realized they would be half the price of the liquid. Instead of costing us $420 per year, it is $210 per year. Since IBM pays four-fifths and we pay only one-fifth, the liquid was actually costing a total of $2,100/year; so using the pills instead saves a thousand dollars per year. The other advantage was that the pills constituted one-eighth of the total daily dose, and thus were given every three hours. The morphine solution was one-sixth of the total daily dose, given every 4 hours. More frequent doses in smaller amounts help preserve a nearly constant level in the blood, and nearly constant pain protection.*

*Tina gets five other prescription medications at various times of the day and six feedings throughout the day with a balanced nutritional fluid. She also receives cranberry juice and yogurt, along with a host of vitamins and minerals. She is in robust health, needed if she has to fight off viruses, for which there is little available effective medication.*

*All of this is kept track of with "charting," listing of each item, its time of ingestion, day by day, the nurses initialing what they have given. A similar set of documents chart the treatments, from bathing, to diaper-changing, to care for the gastric tube site to care for the tracheostomy site, etc.*

*Frequent monitoring of crucial vital signs—blood pressure, pulse rate, blood oxygen saturation, heart rate, respiration rate and volume—has helped us catch incipient infections rapidly. Still, an attack of pneumonia once developed within only a few hours, and we had to call 911 and the emergency medical technicians to rush her to the hospital, forty-five minutes away.*

*Intravenous antibiotics given through a triple-lumen catheter placed in her upper chest, saved her life. A couple of other times, intravenous lines threaded from her arm to a major vein in the chest were sufficient. The irritation of those veins that occurred at that time means that the next time, we will have to re-install a port surgically. It all gets a bit scary.*

*Several doctors have told us she has been receiving exceptional care at home. We call it TLC, "Tina-loving care."*

## NARCOTICS MANAGEMENT

**To keep track of the use of liquid morphine,** we weighed the container on a scale sensitive to tenths of a gram and followed the weight changes over time, comparing with the expected usage. We let the nurses know, informally, that we were keeping track of this.

**When we switched to using pills for the morphine doses, we ran out a week early one time.** We suspected that they had been taken by one of our nurses who had recently had a painful operation. We noted it in the communication book, but did not accuse anybody. After that, we put a limited amount of the pills, about a week's worth, by the nursing station in the home and stored the rest upstairs out of reach.

In the eighth year of her care, we found the patient was not feeling pain when the morphine dose was missed. We reduced the dosing about 20% every month and weaned her off morphine successfully.

## SHIFT NOT COVERED

**For the first time in a decade or so, we recently had a shift not fully covered by the nursing staff.** The nurse scheduled to work that overnight shift (10 p.m. to 8 a.m.) called in the early afternoon to say she did not feel well and was calling other nurses to seek a replacement. In the evening, **she called around 7 p.m. to say she was being admitted to the hospital and had been unable to get any of the nurses she called to respond.** We called the few nurses who might have been able to help, but they could not or would not, even when the pay was doubled for the shift. Finally, the nurse who worked to 10 p.m. agreed to stay to midnight and our head nurse agreed to come at 4 a.m. before she went to her day job. Both got paid double time, although each would have done this for us without that. Subsequently, one of the two was given more scheduled hours, as she had been seeking. **Two family members, one a retired nurse, handled the four hours not covered.**

## *OUTSIDE SUPPORT (COOPER, 2011)*

*"God helps those who help themselves." Let's hope so. More often it seems it is, "God help those who help themselves" because few others will do so.*

*The Multiple Sclerosis Society Support Group in Mt. Kisco (near our Bedford Hills place), c. 1985, was pleasant and encouraging.*

Friendships developed there that lasted years. Still, the newly diagnosed seemed not really happy to see the wheelchair-bound members. Too scary. Cognitive losses can create complications. The more you might benefit from such a group, the less able you are to be involved, and perhaps the less willing the group members are to be involved with you.

In April 2011, I received a card from the National Multiple Sclerosis Society's New York City/Southern New York Chapter, inviting us to register for support groups, one or more of sixty possible choices, to meet for 90 minutes at a session in one of the five boroughs of New York City, some seventy miles south of us. The front cover lists these 17 of the 60, none of which seemed likely to be worth the trek to the city....To be less critical, I might have found worthwhile the "Caregiver" or "Cognitive" or "Stress" groups, had they been nearer to me.

If you choose a country setting to "get away from it all," you must not be surprised if you have gotten a bit too far.

Our friends at Ledgewood Commons (Wendy and Zane, Ruth and Mal) were good company and remained our friends ever since, real psychological support. Wendy's piece in the section at end of the book describes the kind of emotional support that she and Tina gave each other. Ruth was kind enough to accompany Tina and me to church and ended up converting from Judaism to Christianity, with Tina's sponsorship. Zane and Mal and I have remained good friends, and their visits to us usually include a walk around Lake Osiris and the settling of the political and economic affairs of state, nation, and world.

Emails help, too. We have a few steady e-correspondents.

"A friend in need is a friend indeed." That must mean that someone who helps you when you need it is truly a friend. It can't mean that one is more attractive as a friend when needy. Our friends have had a mixed record. Types of support include calls, letters, visits, holiday cards and presents. Some have come through. Some have not.

Neighbors have helped occasionally, but we can't reciprocate, and we do not request it. Sometimes the coming and going of our nurses inconveniences neighbors, but they do not complain. We do appreciate it and thank them warmly.

How about relatives? By the time MS gets truly difficult, after one is 40 or 50, parents are often too old, perhaps no longer alive or are absorbed in the problems they and their other children have. Tina's parents made several monetary gifts to us, representing 10 to 20 percent of our income in those years. The trust fund in their wills represents another few years of income, should it be needed for Tina's welfare. Very generous and much appreciated. Tina's brother and his wife and their children have visited on the day after Christmas each year, driving from her parents' home in Delaware, and giving us nice gifts, including a microwave oven for our kitchen and a flat-screen HDTV for Tina's bedroom. We appreciate it. Her relationship with her sister has long been less warm, so little is expected there.

IBM has been wonderful. We are thankful for all their help. We wish them continued prosperity. Obamacare has us worried, as some companies are choosing to dump their obligations onto the public plan. Such a plan is not going to cover our in-home care 24 hours per day. [IBM created a special program for people needing catastrophic care.]

*After my mother cracked a pelvic bone, we were able to transfer her here from the hospital after a few days. Medicare provided a half-dozen physical therapist visits, after which they stopped, my mother having been "treated," though not greatly improved. My sister has been a big help. Two of my three brothers have contributed to a portion of the added costs.*

*In talking with our staff members, I learn a common story: one child carries most of the responsibility of caring for parents; the others do not. We've done better than that.*

*Granted, if you marry someone, you are taking your chances, "for better or worse, for richer or poorer, in sickness and in health." If you choose to create children, you are signing up for decades of responsibility.*

*We do think, Tina and I, that children have a responsibility, an obligation, from love and duty, to assist their parents in times of need. We hope ours will not have to be called on to sacrifice for us.*

## EXPECT MORE, GET MORE?

We almost entitled this section, "Expect less. Get less. Care less." Expecting less helps shield us from disappointment. Lowered expectations often lead to worse results. Poor results need to be faced stoically. Better:

**Expect more.** Doing so makes you work harder, more optimistically, toward your goals. Others often try to live up to our expectations. Low expectations produce worse behavior. Expecting that another person will treat you unfairly can make that person inclined to treat you less well.

**Get more.** Not only does positive thinking improve our mood, it seems to attract what we are seeking. This "law of attraction" doesn't always work, but it probably does improve our chances. Yet:

**Care less.** We all prefer positive outcomes. If we let outcomes control our happiness, however, we are vulnerable to unhappiness when things do not go our way. Kipling advised that we meet triumph and disaster stoically, and "treat these two imposters just the same." Imposters? Some defeats are to our benefit: "Every knock is a boost." Some victories are Pyrrhic, costing more than they are worth, encouraging us to go in a wrong direction thereafter.

**"Hope for the best and prepare for the worst." Harness positive thoughts, but "keep your powder dry."** For example, IBM announced in August 2013 that it was moving its retirees, like me, from their generous medical plan to Medicare plus partially subsidized supplements. For many, the change was neutral or beneficial. For Tina and me, it would be disastrous, falling far short of the hundreds of thousands of dollars a year that IBM has been providing for Tina's round-the-clock skilled nursing care the prior nine years. After contacting IBM, I scurried around, planning the depletion of our savings, our retirement funds, and money from our two families, preparing for the worst, while hoping IBM would make an exception for exceptional cases.

**In mid-November 2013, we learned that Tina's in-home skilled nursing care would continue to be covered fully. IBM had listened to the concerns of its retirees who were in special situations, and the corporation has modified its plans. Our response: "Thank God. Thank IBM. Thank God for IBM." Our**

**Thanksgiving came a week early.**

When we were informed originally that IBM would not be covering Tina's in-home nursing care, we were advised by friends to pursue legal remedies, to fight. The alternative was to expect that, once aware of situations such as ours, IBM would do the right thing, as it did. Litigating might have been useless or even counter-productive.

# CHAPTER 6

# HOW? PREVENTING, PRESCRIBING, CHARTING, EXPLAINING, TRAVELING, HOSPITALIZATIONS, INFECTION AND CONTAMINATION CONTROL, HIPAA, NURSING CARE PLAN

## PREVENTING INFECTIONS: FLU SHOTS (COOPER, 2011)

*A major threat to quadriplegic patients like Tina is infection, especially respiratory infection and, secondarily, bedsores. If Tina gets the flu, certain antiviral medicines may help, but basically she is on her own—her immune system must create the antibodies that destroy the viruses.*

*Each fall, flu vaccinations are made available to combat the current version of flu, which is different every year. In 2009, a second version, H1N1, became a threat as well.*

*Tina and I each get vaccinated. For people in their 60s, as we are, it reduces our risk of catching the flu by roughly 50 percent.*

We require our nurses to get the shots as a condition of employment, made clear in the interviews we do in selecting new hires. This reduces their risk by 50 percent or a bit more, except that some of them are in contact with large populations of institutional patients who are more likely than most to catch the flu.

In 2010, there was controversy surrounding the safety of the H1N1 vaccine, which controversy seemed to me to be overblown. Regardless, we required this second flu shot, not for the benefit of the nurses, but for the benefit of Tina. Nursing means you take certain responsibilities and some added risks, for example, you drive to work when the roads are slippery. Four of our nurses strung us along several months, not indicating they would not get the H1N1 shots. When they did not get the shots after a month's warning of our deadline, they were fired.

## *PREVENTING INFECTIONS: BEDSORES*

Your skin protects you from infection. Remove even a modest fraction of it and microbes will overwhelm your immune system and kill you. Antibiotics can wipe out some of these organisms, but some have evolved to be multiple-drug-resistant strains that we cannot yet defeat.

Lying in bed (or sitting) motionless keeps pressure on portions of the skin near the supporting bones. Blood to these areas is not supplied or removed in normal amounts, so cells begin to die. Altering the patient's position frequently can prevent this. Urine and fecal matter can irritate the skin, making it more likely to fail. Sliding associated with being moved can exert shear forces that can tear the skin. Once such a sore, a bedsore, develops, the patient is at risk for systemic infection and death; thus, bedsores must be prevented, and treatment started at the first sign of a developing problem.

We had one such sore during Tina's paraplegic period (1994-2004) and one during her current period of quadriplegia (post 2004). The first was due to inadequate attention by a home health aide and me. We should have changed her position more frequently and taken greater pains to keep her clean and dry. The second bedsore resulted during hospitalization, with unusual urinary and bowel incontinence as contributing factors.

At home we have taken many steps to prevent bedsores. We have an air mattress with a checkerboard pattern of air pockets: when the "black" squares are up, the "red" are down and vice-versa, thanks to the action of an air pump that every few minutes changes from inflating one air path and suctioning the other, to the reverse. We also put her on her side a total of a few hours each day. Being placed on her side is less than optimal for Tina, because she cannot rest as well or see the TV as well, but it works out, especially during daytime naps and some periods in the overnight shift.

Our staff has told me horror stories of fist-size bedsores down to the bone on nursing home patients who received inadequate care. By that stage the sores are deadly. Too many patients, too few staff, poor morale among the staff all can contribute. Once a bedsore starts to develop, it is admittedly a challenge to reverse.

Christopher Reeve was the well-known actor (Superman) rendered quadriplegic by the severing of his spinal cord in an equestrian accident in 1995, the year after Tina became bedridden. We closely followed developments in his case. Until 2004, he *wrote and spoke as though he believed his spinal injury would someday be cured. That year he stated that he had lost that faith; bedsores recurred, despite presumably the best of care, and he died from the infection or from a reaction to the antibiotic given to treat it. Small, but deadly are bedsores.*

*We care for Tina's skin very, very diligently.*

**Bedsores, also referred to as "ulcers" or "decubitus ulcers" develop because of lack of blood flow to the skin tissues that are pressed between bony prominences and relatively hard bedding or chair surfaces or because of shear forces from sliding contact between the skin and such surfaces.** In her treatise for Continuing Medical Education for nurses, *Treating Pressure Ulcers and Chronic Wounds,* Maryann Mamou (2014) goes into great detail. She cites the Centers for Medicare and Medicaid Services (CMS) support for her statement that **"a pressure ulcer can develop in at-risk patients within 2 to 6 hours of the onset of pressure."**

**Such sores are serious. "There is a 2 to 6 times greater mortality risk for patients who develop pressure ulcers.** In acute-care hospitals, patient risk for acquiring a pressure ulcer is estimated to range from 14% to 20%." (Mamou, 2014) Indeed, during our younger patient's 100-day stay in the critical care unit, she quickly acquired such ulcers on her heels. Immobility raises the risk greatly. Mamou (2014) cites research showing **"At any given time, 17% to 39% of the spinal cord injured population has a pressure ulcer."** Once one develops, it often recurs, "between 40% and 80% of patients who have had pressure ulcers will develop another one."

The sores can range from Deep Tissue Injury through Stages 1 to 4 in increasing degrees of seriousness. Any indication of a bedsore should trigger remedial action, including increased frequency of change of position, upgrade in mattress design or materials, additional padding and bandaging at the site. The availability of help in treating and transporting the patient will influence the choice of treatments as well. While the development of such sores suggests inadequate care, this is by no means always the case. Elderly patients, especially, may have such fragile skin that even skilled nursing treatment is insufficient to prevent such sores. Patients with cognitive deficits will be unlikely to be able to care for themselves.

Mamou (2014) notes "Many respiratory problems can lead to wound development." This makes sense, as a major factor is inadequate oxygen supply to the tissues at the site, accelerating damage and retarding healing. Steroid use can slow tissue repair, as well. It follows that cardiovascular deficiencies can also accelerate development of the sores and impair healing.

Gastrointestinal problems complicate matters (Mamou, 2014): not only does reduced nutrition slow healing, but the presence of loose stools or even diarrhea causes chemical damage to the skin. Similarly, efforts must be made to keep the skin clean and dry, difficult where incontinence is encountered or where the patient is dependent on disposable undergarments. Too little water has its own negative effect (Mamou, 2014): "Dehydration impairs wound healing by decreasing the blood volume available to transport oxygen and nutrient to healing wounds."

Diabetes raises blood sugar levels and impairs the immune response, thus slowing healing. Obesity puts added pressure at the contact point, and fat tissues are poorly supplied with blood vessels. Information on wound assessment and wound healing is of importance to the nursing staff, less so to the manager. **The most common wounds are "partial-thickness wounds," and (Mamou, 2014) "the most important consideration with partial thickness wounds is to keep the area moist and clean. It is important to remember that a dry cell is a dead cell."** This goes against one's initial thinking: if moisture can contribute to causing the wound, why would it be beneficial? Apparently, the key is protecting the sore from the irritating moisture of urine or damp feces.

Managers should expect that dressing changes will be accompanied by cleanings. "The Agency for Health Care Research and Quality **(AHRQ) recommends that all pressure ulcers be cleaned when first diagnosed and then with every dressing change."** (Mamou, 2014) The goal is to remove loose skin and prevent the growth of bacteria. Normal saline is fine for cleaning, squirted with a syringe, perhaps with a wound-cleansing agent. Dilute bleach or dilute iodine can be used for disinfection, although potentially irritating.

**Mamou (2014) notes that pain management is important.** Analgesic can be given about half an hour before the treatments. Certain elements, such as dressing removal, should be done at a pace acceptable to the patient. "Tape should be avoided on fragile skin."

**Wound dressings** provide cushioning and a barrier to microbes but must both wick moisture from the surface, yet not make it too dry. A nurse with a wound-care specialization is likely to be needed for all but the least severe cases.

This treatise by Mamou we highly recommend for nurses and managers involved in a situation involving wound care. It is available as an ebook from Amazon.

## DOCTOR TRIPS

*We see a pulmonologist four times a year, a throat surgeon four times a year, a general practitioner as needed, typically several times a year. If something is amiss, there will be tests and scans, hither and yon. We bring our most recent records. We record the results of the visit in a book dedicated to doctor visits.*

*Each trip requires the life-support equipment. Each trip is an adventure, because if the specialized van breaks down some-where, we'll have major trouble. The van's lift requires electric power, without which Tina is trapped in the van. If the van's doors jam, the same problem results. Even if we get her out, what next? Call 911 and transfer her to a stretcher and take her home. Don't forget to bring the cell phone.*

*The consequences get more serious if we are brought to a halt during a summer trip. Heat is very hard on MS patients, as it aggravates the deficiencies in the insulating properties of the myelin covering the nerves. In the winter, cold is the threat. We try to schedule most of our trips for the spring and fall, the more temperate seasons.*

## DOCTOR TRIP FROM HECK

*The doctor trip from hell would be one where our special van breaks down on a lonely road in the winter or the summer, with an electrical failure. No heat, no air-conditioning, no power lift for entrance or exit from the van, with Tina stuck inside. As I write this section, on April 25, 2011, we had just had a some-what-less-than-hellish trip.*

*The multi-specialty doctors' practice in Middletown is about twenty miles away, typically a forty-minute ride, plus loading and unloading time. We allocate an hour each way. For this trip, we had originally scheduled back-to-back appointments with two doctors in the group, a pulmonologist and a new gastro-enterologist, to save us from having to make two trips. A few days previously, we were told we had to postpone one of the appointments, because Medicare does not pay for two doctor visits to the same practice on the same day. We put off the pul-monologist for a few days.*

*The van's motor started up well, despite not having been used for a few days. The horn was strangely anemic. The power lift rose more slowly than usual in getting Tina into the van and descended more slowly in delivering her to the doctors' parking lot. An electrical problem? Stay tuned.*

*We waited almost an hour for the gastroenterologist. When we saw him—presentable, articulate, speaking rather good English, though a bit too softly for my poor hearing—it became clear that Tina's feeding tube was not going to be changed then and there, as we thought it would be. No, no. You can't have fed her within five hours of the procedure (which itself is often done by nurses and takes about five minutes). No one had warned us of this. Furthermore, they had no gastric tubes on hand. You have to bring your spare, then they use it and give you a prescription for one or two more. No one had told us this, either.*

When I explained the inconvenience of making two trips, the doctor informed me about the Medicare reimbursement rules, emphasizing that he would not lie for us and claim we had come a different day. Charming. I might have said I would not lie for him and tell someone else that I thought his practice was well run, but I did not. I'm more charming than he is, surpassing a low standard. We used this man because his predecessor gastro kept us waiting a couple of hours without a warning of any kind. What is it with the gastro guys?

After making a new appointment for a week later, we packed up our gear to take our van home. I turned on the ignition — and nothing happened. No gauges moved, no radio came on, certainly no starter motor was motivated. Dead. We tried jump-starting, with the help of the kindness of strangers. No luck. I called AAA. The van's electrical system was too complex for local garages, because of the power-lift modifications for the wheelchair. We called an ambulance and got Tina into it, transferring her from wheelchair to stretcher and folding up the wheelchair to squeeze it into the vehicle. We had wanted an ambulette (wheelchair, not stretcher) service, which would take us all and leave Tina in her chair, but the listing in the Yellow Pages was not sufficiently clear.

Much waiting ensued. Tina, our nurse, and I all were patient. We were in the temperature-controlled waiting area of the office building containing the medical practice, safe and sound. We had two oxygen bottles with us. Nothing really bad happened. Of course, nearly a thousand dollars in ambulance and towing fees were put on the credit card. It's only money. Better yet, it's only plastic.

*In a few days, we were scheduled to return to the same practice, this time for a pulmonary check-up. We could hardly wait.*

*Postscript: We junked that van and bought another, newer, used van, one whose exit access was not dependent on electrical power, so that we could get Tina out of it even without battery power.*

## HOSPITALIZATIONS

*During the seven years since Tina's crisis, we have had an additional few hospitalizations, generally for a week each, and generally associated with an infection of some kind. Respiratory infections are the most dangerous, but urinary tract infections can also become systemic and life-threatening.*

*If the infective agent is a virus, not much can be done to fight it except to support the patient as her immune system battles to save her life. Combating secondary bacterial infection is often required, too. A bacterial pathogen is likely to be susceptible to antibiotic treatment. A mild broad-spectrum antibiotic might suffice, though often one needs a stronger drug tailored to the specific type of organism, Gram-negative or Gram-positive, staphylococcus or pseudomonas, etc. Medicine that can be given orally (by gastric tube, in Tina's case) is more easily administered than medicine that needs to be given intravenously. In Tina's case, several such IV treatments have left her arm and foot veins too fragile. That's why a chest-level port will be needed.*

*When she is hospitalized, we have our own nurses accompany her, doing as little or as much as the hospital staff is comfortable* with. *This is expensive, as our insurance does not cover this second layer of nurses; but it assures that her special needs are understood and receive attention. It provides continuity of care for her and continuity of employment for the nurses.*

## FIGHTING FOR YOUR PATIENT

**You will want to get as familiar with your patient's diagnosis, treatment, and prognosis as you can.** While the patient is in the hospital or at home, you will need to keep alert and to ask questions. During the 100 days my [DWC's] wife was in the Critical Care Unit of our Orange County [NY] Regional Medical Center, I did just this, as described in our book, *Ting and I,* in the Foreword written by our principal doctor on the case, Richard F. Walker, MD:

*Intensive care specialists learn to cope with the possibility of bad outcomes, in part, by de-personalizing the patient into a series of physiologic challenges, much as the combat soldier might resist making very close friends when the chance of death is ever-present. The battle for life, then, consists of attempts by the medical staff to raise blood oxygen, combat infection, preserve nutrition and urinary output and avoid hospital-acquired infection.*

*The physician thus runs the risk of partially replacing the patient as the object of care by worrying about the frequency of reportable iatrogenic complications, medico-legal risks and reimbursement considerations.*

*Dr. Jerome Groopman in his excellent book* **How Doctors Think** *describes the biases and decision-making consequences of* *such distractions, as well as the dangers of projecting one's own concept of meaningful existence onto others. He specifically singles out the important role of the patient or patient-advocate in refocusing the physician on what is objectively possible and beneficial.*

*Such a bias crept into my own thinking as my mounting feelings of hopelessness at returning Tina to a level of function worthy of the effort were rejected by Doug. His exhortations for better care were often viewed by me as selfishly motivated and without sufficient regard for the burden and suffering the illness was creating for Tina. My attempts to gauge her feelings during Doug's infrequent absences from her bedside revealed that her goals mirrored his. I attributed her attitude to a desire not to hurt or disappoint him, or to stereotypical Asian stoicism.*

*Doug tirelessly directed the attention of the health care team to seemingly trivial aspects of her care, asking detailed questions and demanding satisfactory answers, even occasionally suggesting changes in her care plan. My periodic annoyance, hopefully not always apparent, served to refocus my attention away from the pathophysiology and back to Tina. What I did not initially realize was that Doug's persistence was improving his wife's care.*

Being human, doctors and nurses respond to encouragement and criticism, and your attitude will affect theirs. Up to a point, the more interest you show, the more involved they will be. Any virtue can be overdone, however, and one must gauge whether you are risking raising hostility rather than improving care.

# YOUR NURSES, YOUR DOCTOR, THEIR HOSPITAL

**Recently (February 2016), our 71-year-old quadriplegic patient became ill, running a fever (rectal, body core temperature of 104°F), and she was taken by ambulance to the Emergency Room of the regional medical center, a new facility built a few years ago, located some 20 miles from our home.**

Much had changed since she was at the same hospital three years ago: there are no longer restrictions on visiting hours. Patients and their visitors are allowed to use cell phones now. In general, an effort was made to make it convenient for patients and their families.

**As is our practice, we had our nurses accompany her while going to and from and while staying at the hospital, even though our insurance does not cover doing that.**

Having our own nurses there has the advantage that errors made by the hospital staff are likely to be picked up and corrected. In one case, a hospital nurse inadvertently and unobtrusively left a tourniquet on our patient's foot after drawing a blood sample. A while afterward, our own nurse noticed that one foot was different in color from the other, and when our nurse investigated further, she found that indeed the tourniquet had been left on. She removed it. The first two nights, our patient did not sleep well. On the third day, our nurse noted that the hospital staff had not given our patient her nighttime Ativan anti-anxiety medication. When this was done on the third night, after the omission was brought to the attention of the hospital staff, our patient slept much better.

In some instances, our nurses were able to accelerate some aspects of the care, either by helping out or by calling her needs to the attention of the hospital staff.

**As a general rule, it seems likely that having one's own nurses to help and observe improves the care the patient receives, especially where the patient has problems communicating or understanding, as was true here.**

We tell our nurses to do as much or as little as the hospital is comfortable having them do. We found that the hospital staff was very cooperative with our nurses, something we greatly appreciated.

It can be a bit boring for our nurses to have less to do while on hospital duty with our patient, but perhaps the change of scene and the fact that they're getting paid without having direct responsibility offsets the disadvantage of possible boredom.

Communicating to our staff the whereabouts of the patient in this situation is a little complicated, but cell phone calls and texting allowed us to coordinate the nurses' attendance, first at the hospital and then back home right after our patient returned.

**In talking with the doctors to try to get an unambiguous diagnosis, I found there was a lot of ambiguity.** The chest x-rays which could indicate whether or not there was pneumonia were complicated by the presence of a bit of post-mastectomy prosthesis material placed two decades earlier in the area in front of the lower right lobe of the lung, and initially a haziness seen there was interpreted as pneumonia, but later this region was ignored after the issue of a prosthesis was raised. Of course, ignoring that region would miss signs of pneumonia that happened to be there.

**Using two antibiotics intravenously, the hospital rapidly returned our patient's vital signs to her normal levels, essentially overnight.** The next few days, these vital signs remained relatively normal, and we waited for results from the analyses of urine and blood samples taken the first day.

Our patient entered the hospital Sunday evening, and she was cleared by the infectious disease specialist MD to leave the hospital Wednesday evening, which we did. **It never became clear what the cause of her fever was, but the infectious disease specialist indicated it was probably pneumonia, which, if viral, was cured by the patient's immune system, and if bacterial, was eradicated by vancomycin and Zosyn antibiotics. Interestingly, hospital personnel advised us to get our patient discharged as soon as it was safe to do so, as hospital-acquired (nosocomial) infections were common.**

Our patient came home with a revised list of prescriptions, including prescriptions for yet a third and fourth antibiotic, Levaquin and Macrodantin. Two days later, we reviewed the revised prescriptions with our own family doctor, who concurred in the antibiotic additions, but who mostly decided to retain the doses and timing that we originally had for her other medications, rather than adopt the somewhat different recommendations of the hospitalist.

**Hospitals prefer to use their doctors rather than yours.** When our patient was admitted to the hospital, we requested that her pulmonologist be involved in consulting about her care.

Although it was decided that she would be admitted to the hospital by the authority of the hospitalist, we were given to understand that her pulmonologist would be consulted.

He did not come the following day, Monday, so on Tuesday morning, I [DWC] drove to his office a mile or so away from the hospital, and I talked with his secretary, as he was out of town. She indicated that **he was aware that we wanted him involved, but the hospital had raised a bureaucratic objection to this.** I immediately returned to the hospital, talked with the patients' advocate department, who were very accommodating, and it was quickly arranged that our pulmonologist be invited to consult, which he did that evening and the next day. So, while the hospital initially made it difficult for our private doctor to be involved, their appeal process worked quite well.

By the time our pulmonologist arrived, the patient's vital signs were nearly normal, as were her lung sounds, and there had been no clear indication of pneumonia on the chest x-rays, so he hypothesized other causes, none of which explained the 104-degree rectal thermometer reading Sunday night, nor its rapid reduction after the administration of IV antibiotics.

While at the hospital, we met the pulmonologist who had been involved with our patient's care 12 years previously, and she seemed to be readily available there, so the next time we may use her rather that our private pulmonologist. That plan suggests that we establish a continuing relationship with the hospital's MD, having our patient see her perhaps twice a year, as we were doing with the other pulmonologist who had difficulty getting to the hospital when we needed him.

In general, we were quite satisfied with the care provided by the hospital, and their cooperativeness and their willingness to have our patient leave after a short stay, to help reduce the risk of her picking up germs from other patients.

Another plus for the hospital's practices is that they made the results of all the tests done available, at a website that we could access once we set up a user identification name and a password. We were able to print out the results and bring a subset of these to our family doctor two days later when we wanted to discuss the wisdom of changing the prescriptions.

# INFECTION CONTROL

Homes, as well as hospitals, have got to maintain strict practices if infection of the patient or the caregivers is to be avoided. This brief presentation cannot cover all important aspects of infection control, but it should help you understand the major issues.

The basic elements of infection are viruses, bacteria, and fungi (yeast, *etc.*). Viruses are not quite alive, but they capture the mechanisms of a cell to enable themselves to be replicated, often damaging the host; flu and HIV viruses are familiar. Bacteria are single-celled organisms that can replicate on their own but use the host to enhance their growth; gastro-intestinal ailments and skin wound infections are typically due to bacteria. Fungi are single-celled or multi-celled organisms that, like bacteria, feed off the host; they spread by producing spores; "yeast" infections are due to fungi.

A systematic approach to infection control looks at the following items:

**Sources: Infected people are the major hazard.** Post notices that people with colds should not come in the house or the room. That includes nurses, unless they are wearing respiratory equipment, not just masks, but equipment that completely filters what they exhale (e.g., through a HEPA filter, a High-Efficiency Particulate Air filter, an "absolute filter" 99.9+% efficient). Face masks allow leakage around the edges in contact with the skin and are usually made of low-efficiency filter material. They do prevent spit from speaking or coughing from becoming airborne. Unfortunately, the patient may come home from the hospital with an infection ("nosocomial" or "iatrogenic"), perhaps "colonized," quite possibly a danger to the staff and family.

**Transmission: Coughing, talking, sneezing, as well as shedding from exposed skin,** make the organisms airborne, allowing them to travel to the patient, unless the patient is breathing air which is filtered by an absolute filter. **Direct surface contact** occurs when the patient is touched by someone who is contaminated. **Indirect surface contact** occurs when a contaminated person touches a surface that is subsequently touched by the patient or by someone who touches the patient. **Instruments** brought into contact with the patient can carry infectious agents ("germs"), which are particularly dangerous when the skin is broken or the probe goes inside the body. **Food and drink and medicines** can bring dangerous biological agents, as well, although the stomach is not sterile and its acidity generally handles the destruction of most organisms without allowing illness.

**Barriers:** For **airborne transmission,** one can try to direct clean air toward the patient and against the flow of contaminated air; pharmaceutical and microelectronics manufacturing

**cleanrooms are kept at higher pressures than their environ-
ments, and the pressure in a ventilator mask can be set so as
not to become a slight vacuum when the patient inhales,** so
that it is always at a "positive pressure" with respect to the air
in the room. **Contact transmission** from caregivers and others
is reduced by **the use of disposable gloves,** which themselves
must be kept clean or replaced frequently. Sometimes, a second
pair is worn over the first, so that a change can be made readily when the outer pair become contaminated. Caregivers and
visitors should **wash their hands thoroughly** before and after
coming in contact with the patient, preferably with an antibacterial soap. Ideally, objects brought into contact with the patient would be clean and sterile, but in practice **those objects
making external contact are cleaned and disinfected** (e.g., with
alcohol/water or vinegar/water solutions), rather than **sterilized**
(e.g., with bleach or iodine solutions or submersion in boiling
water), which is **appropriate for internal contact or contact
with broken skin. Wounds and sores are protected with antibiotic ointments or petroleum jelly and** with impermeable
coverings such as bandages, except where exposure to the air
through a gauze dressing is prescribed instead.

**Removal:** Although little can be done to remove airborne agents
once inhaled, **those that settle on the skin can be removed
with washing and disinfecting or even using sterilizing solutions.** Where cuts are involved, the value of sterility may be
offset by the possible chemical harshness of a sterilizing agent,
leading to the use instead of various "antibacterial" solutions
that include soap and anti-microbial chemicals, or simply soap,
or an alcohol/water solution and rubbing with the fabric containing it. Harmful chemicals that are ingested are sometimes
removed by encouraging vomiting, using an emetic liquid, but

one rarely knows that a liquid with dangerous germs has recently been ingested.

**Hardening the target:** To **make the patient less susceptible to infection** is a major goal of the maintenance of general good health, including optimal nutrition and adequate sleep. Viral infections must be defeated by the patient; **vaccinations** help prepare the immune system for this battle. For the elderly, however, flu shots are often only 50% efficient, and for younger people only somewhat better. **We require our nurses to get vaccinated against the flu, as do the patients and the family.**

**Remedy:** If the patient becomes ill, **the causal organism is determined and medicine prescribed, if available.** As noted, little can be done about most **viruses** once they are active, except to maintain the patient's general health. For a **urinary tract infection**, a common ailment in chronic illness situations, a urine sample is taken and tested against available drugs, a **"culture and sensitivity" test**, which will indicate to which antibiotics the organism is "sensitive," meaning susceptible. **Secretions from the lung, sputum,** can be analyzed similarly for the same purpose. An infected wound will be treated by a broad-spectrum antibiotic cream or ointment, often after receiving wiping with a disinfectant or a sterilizing agent in a pad. These infections can lead to more general, **systemic, infections** which **have to be caught immediately (by noting elevated temperature, pulse rate, respiration rate) and treated with antibiotics,** administered orally, by gastric tube, intravenously, or by intra-muscular injections, as ordered by the doctor.

# CONTAMINATION CONTROL

The considerations for contamination control are similar to those for infection control, except that **it would be unusual for a contaminating chemical to reach the patient in a dose large enough to cause illness. Sources** need to be identified and eliminated or minimized. **Transmission** through the air is prevented by the use of clean air flowing toward the source rather than from it or by the use of filters, **filtered air supply**, and facemasks for the patient and caregivers. **Face masks** generally will reduce the inhaled concentration of airborne solids and liquids (**aerosols**) but not eliminate them and rarely are they effective on **toxic gases**, should any be present.

**Spills of liquids and powders** need to be cleaned up carefully and thoroughly. A spill should be absorbed in a wiper that is then discarded; next, the area is rinsed with clean water, and that water absorbed and that wiper discarded, too. Wipe from the cleanest toward the dirtiest, from the driest toward the wettest. Gloves should be used. **Using a damp wipe on the patient's skin** will transfer some skin oils and salts from caregiver to patient, unless the wipe is held in a glove. **Liquids or powders spilled onto the floor represent a hazard from reduced traction** for the staff, leading to slips and falls. Even a dry cloth or paper on the floor can represent a hazard; we lost a nurse for three months after she slipped on a dryer anti-static sheet in our laundry room. [She should not have dropped it, should have picked it up, should have not stepped on it, but "should" doesn't mean "didn't."]

**Removal of contaminants** from the patient is normally done with soap and water or alcohol and water, again with a gloved hand holding a clean, damp wipe. Removal is completed when the surface is wiped dry.

## HIPAA CONTROL

This section alerts you to the risk of running afoul of the Federal Health Information Portability and Accountability Act of 1996, HIPAA. **Basically, you want to keep medical information confidential**. Grant (2014) describes the mechanisms necessary to achieve and maintain compliance. He represents a company that offers services of this kind: the Compliancy Group, LLC. "LLC" for "Limited Liability Corporation" means they have taken steps to incorporate and limit their liability, just in case. In case of what? In case someone takes their advice, gets in trouble with the Feds, and tries to blame Grant and Group. They offer The Guard, to control the audit process: "regulatory review, risk analysis, risk management, document management, and incident management." You can contact them at info@compliancygroup.com.

A homeowner is not likely to need the Group's services, but is well advised to keep the medical information of the patient restricted to those with what the government calls "need to know." The doctors treating the patient will likely want the protection of signed acknowledgment of their HIPAA policies, restrictions, and practices designed to safeguard patient information.

The seriousness of these HIPAA issues is reflected in the costs of the ebooks on the topic at Amazon. The first 15 in terms of relevance ranged from $1 to $430, with half costing $25 or more.

The manager of nursing care at home should assure that sensitive information is not stored on computers connected to the Internet and that paper copies be carefully handled so as to prevent theft or loss.

# NURSING CARE PLANS

**Nursing care is much more than administering physician-ordered medications and completing assessment sheets. A professional registered nurse also develops care plans for patients. These are guides that identify a patient's medical or emotional condition and difficulty and details scientifically based nursing actions to improve the condition.** Knowing the basis of nursing plans may help in understanding the clinical reasoning, logic, and information that follows in our chapters concerning patient illnesses, treatments, and care considerations for your patient

If you have skilled nursing services providing care for your family member, you may come across **Nursing Care Plans.** While you will not be responsible for formulating plans, implementing the protocols, or generally being involved with them, you should have a basic understanding of what they are and how they are used in nursing.

**A nursing care plan begins with a diagnosis. A nursing diagnosis differs from a medical diagnosis.** A medical diagnosis is formulated using scientific and clinical data to determine a disease process, illness, or injury. A physician uses this diagnosis to plan courses of treatment to minimize or eliminate the medical disorder, such as by prescribing medications and ordering tests.

In nursing, the diagnosis is also determined using assessment and clinical data, and actually quite similar in the end-product, which is to benefit the patient's health. However, **the results of what the patient is experiencing is diagnosed, not the medical ailment.** For example, a medical diagnosis could be "mesothelioma, lung cancer, and surgical removal of a lung lobe." A nursing diagnosis, which depicts the condition or problem the patients exhibits, could be "impaired gas exchange," which is related to the removal of pulmonary tissue and decreased functioning of lung tissue due to the disease process. These directly relate to the patient's inability to oxygenate blood, yet don't specifically relate to the lack of lung tissue or specify a disease. **All nursing diagnoses directly correspond to the patient needs and/or conditions.** Nursing diagnoses begin the care plan after assessment of the patient and diagnosis from those approved by the North American Nursing Diagnosis Association (NANDA).

**The nursing diagnosis is determined by defining characteristics which validate the diagnosis.** They may be both subjective and objective. Subjective characteristics, again using the example noted above, would be difficulty breathing (dyspnea) as in "I can't catch my breath;" chest pain, because the lungs aren't sufficiently expanding; or describing periods of lightheadedness. These are reportable by the patient or family members. **Objective characteristics** are measurable or perceptible by the nurse, such as: **abnormal breath sounds** heard with or without a stethoscope, **thick and tenacious sputum**, **decreased blood oxygen saturation** of less than 92% with supplemental oxygen, **heart rate above normal**, and **confusion and restlessness** due to decreased oxygenation of the brain.

**Outcomes can then be proposed. Outcomes are the positive, measurable benefits and goals expected to be achieved in a specified amount of time by implementing the nursing care**

**plan.** Positive outcomes are evidenced by presenting data and are measurable. **For example, the patient is to have "increased gas exchange within 4 days as evidenced by** decreased dyspnea at rest or exertion, increased sputum production to relieve congestion, increased of level of consciousness, decreased respiratory and heart rate, decreased adventitious breath sounds."

**Once the nursing diagnosis is determined and supported by defining characteristics (the first part) and the outcome is hypothesized (the end result), the actions to get there are proposed and eventually tested by the evidence that the goal was or was not achieved. The path to achieve those goals, stated as outcomes, is then detailed by listing interventions and rationales. Interventions,** very simply stated, are actions: "What I am going to do for the patient." **Rationales** are the reasons why the interventions will benefit the patient: "This will help because...."

**Examples of interventions and rationales** for the patient included **elevating the head of the bed (the intervention)** because it provides increased oxygenation and decreases pressure on the diaphragm, thereby **promoting ease of breathing (the rationale).** Auscultating (listening to) lung sounds and assessment of breathing and respiratory values include noting rate and quality of the respirations every 2 hours; these checks provide positive or negative changes in the patient's condition. **Signs of further decrease in function** would be shallow respirations, nasal flaring, increases in heart rate, and decreases in level of consciousness. These are all further evidence of lack of oxygen due to decreased gas exchange and would indicate further decline. **Giving the patient more fluids** (an intervention) would help to loosen tenacious secretions, and noting input amounts provides indication whether sufficient quantities are being consumed.

**Teaching and assisting the patient with frequent deep breathing exercises and use of incentive spirometer** maximizes expansion of lung tissue including smaller airways. Teaching and assisting patients with splinting their chest and effective coughing when sitting up aids to relieve chest discomfort and maximizes production. These are all examples of nursing interventions based upon a diagnosis of impaired gas exchange. They are intended to treat the condition of the patient—not the disease the patient has.

**The nursing process and nursing care plans are adjustable.** They change and are amended as the patient's condition improves or worsens. **Additionally, nursing care plans do not solely involve the nursing profession.** They are collaborative and involve all aspects of the patient's care-giving team, such as respiratory therapists, physical therapists, physicians, and numerous other professionals involved in the patient's path to well-being.

**A detailed example of such a nursing care plan is given in Appendix 5.**

In the following chapters we turn our attention to managing the nursing care at home for some conditions with which we lack first-hand at-home experience, thus having to rely on the medical literature, our training and our experience in other venues.

**While not all medical conditions, situations, or disease processes can be addressed in depth in this book, the authors felt it was important not to ignore other events and illnesses that**

**your patient may be experiencing.** There are so many illnesses that can occur, that we needed to take a different approach from an illness-specific one. To do so, we decided to use the classification system often used in medical settings for assessments. Within the eleven principal categories will be highlighted some of the more common illnesses. In some cases, as with cancer, several categories are involved. In addition, this section will also speak to the method of assessment and the systemic approach which typically dictates medical practice. As much as possible, this section will follow that system-based approach. **Familiarity with these assessment categories will assist in the understanding and management of nursing care.**

**The Nursing Assessment form used in our home situation is separated according to various systems. This is a standard approach to all nursing documentation.** Assessments are not haphazard comments about the patient. Rather, assessments are a standard method of examining the patient and recording data in a precise manner based upon the function of a particular system.

**Some overlap of findings may occur between systems.** This should not be considered unusual. The body uses individual systems that interact with each other to maintain the body as a unit.

**When one system is failing,** or having difficulty, **the body reacts to try to achieve a functioning that is as normal and balanced as possible** (homeostasis). Perhaps the best way to illustrate this is by a simple analogy: When the mother has the flu, the father steps in and cooks dinner for the family. He doesn't cook as well as mom, usually, but the kids are fed, mom can rest, and he isn't overworked, so he can go to his job in the morning and perform well.

**When the body has a dysfunctional system, the other systems step in and help.** They might not do as well as the ailing system, but, at least temporarily, positive functioning continues. For example: when respiratory function is decreased, the heart rate and therefore the cardiac output (blood flow) increases to deliver oxygenated blood to tissues.

**This cannot continue indefinitely.** The other systems help out, but eventually cannot maintain homeostasis. As in the example above, the increased heart rate tires the heart; it may increase in size, eventually causing cardiac dysfunction, be less able to pump, and/or eventually cease working altogether.

**Monitoring individual systems provides an insight to the operation of the whole body. Adverse changes to more than one system can then alert to multiple system problems, and indicate the need for intervention.**

Discussion in detail of the various body systems resumes with Chapter 10 on the nervous system.

Chapters 7, 8, and 9 cover issues of insurance and medical billing.

# CHAPTER 7

# LONG-TERM CARE INSURANCE

Betty Wilson (2014) presented a comprehensive, yet succinct, description of the whys and wherefores of long-term care insurance. She starts: "...ironically, many of us forget about long-term care insurance, even though, according to statistics, **70% of Americans will need some form of long-term care after the age of 65.**" As Wilson states, "Long-term care includes services offered to people who are suffering from a chronic disease, cognitive impairment, or a disabling condition."

While in our forties, Tina and I [DWC] were able to purchase long-term care insurance for both of us (Cooper, 2011):

*During my IBM employment, the John Hancock Insurance Company got IBM to allow them to offer a special deal for the IBM employees to obtain long-term care insurance. The options had fixed total payouts, with the middle option that we chose being a total of $210,000, several times my annual salary at that time. They could not deny participation due to prior medical conditions, and we were open about Tina's multiple sclerosis, the symptoms of which were mild back then.*

*Five or ten years later, when we met the disability requirements to qualify for weekly supplementation of our home health aide's salary, Hancock started paying about $250 per week to reimburse us. This went on for fourteen years, paying about half to two-thirds of the cost of our aides, who typically worked a thirty-hour to forty-hour week.*

**Home health aides provide "custodial care," the kind of care a dependent infant or disabled or incompetent person needs, without supplying medical care.** They handle the Significant Activities of Daily Living that the patient cannot. Although most people probably get their aides from agencies, we advertised in the paper and obtained aides with certifications that Hancock accepted or had a nurse review their performance and certify that they were qualified without formal credentials.

**Medicaid has significant restrictions on paying for such care, and Medicare rarely pays for home health aides at all.**

Wilson (2014) describes the following "care choices":

- **Care in the home:** "Providers who are eligible to offer home health-care include qualified home health-care agencies or independent care givers who deliver home care, the home of a relative or friend, or a community-based residential facility." One must assure the agency is certified and the care is provided by one or more of the following: nurses, therapists, social workers, certified home health aides or nursing assistants. Family members can sometimes become deemed to be qualified.
- **Care in the community**: Various adult day care centers

and group programs are used to supplement the care obtained at home.

- **Care in an alternate living facility:** "An alternate living facility basically offers ongoing care" outside the home. They offer a wide range of services, and selection will depend on the patient's needs.
- **Care in a nursing home:** This situation provides living quarters and nursing care on a round-the-clock availability.
- **Accessory dwelling units:** Second living spaces in close proximity to the home allow some independence without putting the patient far from the family.
- **Continuing-care retirement communities:** "CCRCs are retirement communities offering more than a single type of housing. They offer different care levels."
- **Hospice care:** for terminally ill patients. Medicare usually covers this.
- **Respite care:** short-term assistance to allow the primary caregiver to rest. Medicare covers up to 5 days of this if you are receiving hospice services.
- Some states have other programs beyond these.

For more information on long-term care insurance, see Wilson (2014) or obtain information from insurers in your state.

# CHAPTER 8

# EMPLOYER'S MEDICAL INSURANCE: OUR EXPERIENCE (Cooper, 2011)

*I [DWC] worked for IBM for a decade, from 1983-1993, and was covered during that time by their Empire Blue Cross/Blue Shield policy at work and for another decade after taking an early retirement buy-out that included their continuing medical coverage. What follows is as brief summary of that experience, along with what happened with the successor insurance companies, MVP, and then United Healthcare, which companies IBM contracted with to manage the medical coverage for some of its retirees.*

## EMPIRE BLUE CROSS / BLUE SHIELD, 1983-2004

*While I was working at IBM, most of our medical costs were quite routine and well covered by their health plan policy.*

*During the 100-days' war against Tina's aspiration-caused pneumonia, from February to June 2004, we ran up roughly a half-million dollars in hospital expenses, covered by IBM's policy with Empire Blue Cross/Blue Shield of New York State. When she returned home, round-the-clock skilled nursing was simi-larly covered, without a problem by Empire BC/BS, whether the billing came from the nursing agency or from me.*

## INSURANCE BLUES: MVP, 2005

*One must sometimes fight one's insurers.*

*At the start of 2005 we were moved by IBM from Empire to MVP. We started round-the-clock skilled nursing care with an agency in June 2004, and I started hiring nurses to fill the gaps in the agency coverage a few months after we began this. By January 2005, I had taken over hiring the nurses, at a higher salary than the agency had been paying, then training and managing them, and billing the insurers for a cost mid-way between what the agency was charging and what the nurses were receiving; I was changing what our actual cost was.*

*MVP wanted more documentation than Empire had required. We sent them reams.*

*MVP wanted to stop paying for the skilled nursing at home, la-beling Tina's need as "custodial care" rather than "skilled nurs-ing care." Custodial care is roughly equivalent to babysitting, which would include giving bottles and making diaper changes. Tina was on a ventilator, fed through a gastric tube, quadriple-gic, and in pain if morphine were not given in proper amounts at proper times. There were about a half-dozen prescription medications to be given at various times during the day and night. The gastric tube needed daily care. The tracheostomy needed daily care.*

*All activities needed to be documented, to assure they were done, to provide continuity of care from shift to shift. We had hospital orders for all this, along with a doctor's orders as well. Still, MVP carped. They planned to stop paying for daytime skilled nursing care. They refused to pay for overnight care.*

*From 10:00 p.m. to 8:00 a.m., through all of 2005, I was the overnight nurse, resting beside Tina, getting up for the administration of medicines, answering over-pressure or under-pressure alarms from the ventilator, suctioning secretions from her trachea, changing her disposable diapers by rolling her carefully on the bed while keeping from hurting her tender wrist joints.*

*I do believe "work is love made real," and this was a labor of love. The loss of sleep was less a problem than was the fear that I would be alone when we lost electrical power, as we do several times each year here, or when she had an emergency condition requiring my immediate attention and my calling for help simultaneously. Evacuating her from a fire would be terribly difficult alone, too. Walking the dog briefly or checking some questionable condition outside meant abandoning her. Not good, not good.*

*We appealed the proposed removal of MVP financial support for the daytime nurses, and we pushed for overnight skilled nursing as well. Two levels of MVP reviewers turned us down. Two levels of IBM reviewers turned us down. An independent outside medical review, our last hope, vindicated our position entirely. Yes, one must sometimes fight.*

*We had started replacing some of the agency nurses as early as August 2004. By January 2005, I believe, we no longer used* *the agency. We started hiring overnight nurses in January 2006. MVP was slow to pay, getting behind a month or two for much of the year. At $25,000 per month, this created a significant cash-flow problem.*

## UNITED HEALTHCARE

*Next, we were switched by IBM to United Healthcare (UHC), the group we are with now. They were less demanding than MVP, and more helpful; but the transition delayed our reimbursements (we pay the nurses, weekly, ourselves) for two or even three months, amounting to $50,000 to $75,000 in arrears. I fear that few other couples would have had the savings we had that let us cover this shortfall. Eventually, UHC caught up, to our relief.*

*Thank you, United Healthcare.*

## THANKS TO IBM

In the decade since 2005, IBM has paid more than five million dollars for Tina's care. My decisions to work for IBM and, ten years later, to take their early-retirement buy-out, paid off for us. We are greatly appreciative. The ten years I worked for IBM proved to be the best working situation I ever had.

# CHAPTER 9

# DIAGNOSING AND REDUCING YOUR MEDICAL BILL
**(from Gross and Cooper, 2015)**

*This chapter consists of various topics, guidance, and suggestions to potentially reduce your medical expenses.*

### How to Cut Your Medical Bills

*Know your rights / be aware of your medical benefits.*

*It is not an easy task to understand your medical bills and the Explanation of Benefits. But to know your rights and be aware of your medical benefits, you must scrutinize your medical insurance policy.*

*Know what you are covered for and what your exclusions are. Exclusions in an insurance policy list what you are not covered for.*

*Call the hospital and medical providers. Check to see what the fees will be. Also check, "What was the doctor's grade for my disease?"*

***Is This Test Required? Why is This Test Required? Save Money!***

*Sometimes, especially if you feel that you are being over-tested or charged too much money for a procedure, ask the medical provider, "What options might be less expensive to get the information you need to accurately diagnose my problem?"*

***If a doctor is recommending a test, it is best to call your health insurance carrier and ask whether the test might require pre-approval.*** *An example is an endoscopy.*

*Make sure your doctor or hospital has insurance pre-approval before the procedure is performed.*

*Also make sure by contacting the insurance carrier that the medical provider has a contract with your insurance carrier. I also recommend that you ask for this in writing. I hear so many cases where the provider's office states that there has been an approval or the medical provider verbally informs you that they have a contract with your health insurance carrier, and they do not.*

*If you are about to have surgery and pre-tests are required before the main procedure, make sure your health insurance carrier has agreed to the services and that they have a contract with the pre-test companies. Location of services and medical provider must both be approved.*

*Ask the provider if you are required to have someone drive you home after the procedure.*

*If you learn that multiple tests are not required, you will save* money. On the other hand **if multiple tests are required, it is best to have them performed on the same day and location.** Many medical providers are against that since they are able to make more money if the procedures are on different dates. One of the major reasons for the Affordable Care Act, ACA, was to require all hospitals and medical providers to share medical information via electronic medical records, hopefully reducing the number of duplicated tests.

Many insurance companies hire an outside company that does the approval for pre-certification.

**If you are informed that the medical provider is not approved, ask your health insurance carrier who the approval company is** and if they if they know which other doctors the pre-cert company might approve.

Perhaps it goes without saying that you will also try to assure yourself of the qualifications of the doctor who you are seeing, to avoid the situation depicted by a cartoonist who depicts one patient saying to another, "Yes—that's my surgeon—the one who cuts himself shaving...."

### Options for the Uninsured and Underinsured

Medicare has an 80/20 agreement; therefore, if you have a hospital bill of $30,000 do you want to be responsible for 20% of the $30,000, which is $6,000? That is the reason why, **if you are able to afford it, it is often best to have either basic Medicare with a supplementary health insurance coverage or one of the Medicare Advantage Plans, which often have rules different from the 80/20 rule.**

***If your employer offers a plan, find out what you are covered for** and determine whether you would want additional health insurance through your spouse or partner. Also, discuss with your and / or your spouse's employer what options are available to you. Sometimes they might have different insurance carriers to choose from or different levels of coverage. If there is no coverage, contact the state to see what it might offer. For example, in New York State, go to https://nystateofhealth.ny.gov/*

***Medicare Advantage Plans** are health plans that are approved by Medicare and provided by private companies. Medicare sets the rules for Medicare Advantage Plans and regulates the private companies who operate the Plans. See our chapter on these plans.*

***Medicare Advantage Plans** cover Medicare Part A and Part B, sometimes including vision and dental care. You pay a copay and/or a deductible; you still pay Medicare premium and might need to also pay an additional premium.*

*Typically you are required to see the plan's network doctors and you cannot buy a Medicare supplement to help pay out-of-pocket expenses.*

*Sometimes it is advantageous to go out of the United States for medical care, but precautions need to be taken.*

***Health Insurance Portability and Accountability Act of 1996: Privacy***

*HIPAA mandates all health insurance companies that are covered entities make the transition to ICD-10. Workmen's compensation and property and casualty insurance companies are not covered entities.*

*For example, I see a new doctor for the first time due to a cold. The procedure code is 99201 (new patient, office visit), the ICD-9 code is 460 and the ICD-10 code is J00, a cold. I go back to the doctor a few days later due to conjunctivitis, the procedure code is 99211, established patient; the ICD-10 code is H10.*

**What this means to all of us is: beginning October 1, 2014, if your diagnosis does not begin with a letter, question your doctor, otherwise your insurance company will deny the claim.**

**Who Is Processing Your Medical Bill?**

**Many hospitals and individual doctors hire outside companies to handle all of their medical bills.** *Either the bill is handled by the medical provider, hospital, doctor, laboratory company or it is sent to an outside medical billing company that is hired by the medical provider.*

*Where do problems occur?*

*The problems occur if the billing company or the medical practice:*

1. *does not handle any of the follow-ups,*
2. *does not submit the bills to your secondary or tertiary insurer,*
3. *is incompetent to bill correctly,*
4. *sends your medical bills to overseas medical billing companies,*

5.  does not have the prior pre-approval for the necessary procedures,
6.  makes errors with pre-authorization, or
7.  if the bills are not submitted within the insurance company's allowed time period.

## How to Decode the Bill?

Most of the bills are now submitted electronically and when done so, the same information that is on a CMS 1500 form is required.

## What To Do With The Bill Once Decoded? Is The Bill Within Reasonable And Customary Charges?

All bills, when paid by Medicare, Medicaid or a commercial health insurance carrier are determined according to procedure codes. Commercial insurers follow Medicare except normally on a higher payout percentage.

Medicare and Medicaid also add a Diagnosis Related Group code, called a DRG code, when determining the payment for hospitalization as an inpatient.

To find the Medicare Allowable Usual, Reasonable and Customary codes, look at the Medicare website. You will find the listings under:

http://www.cms.gov/apps/physician-fee-schedule/

## The Buck Stops Here

*Fight and never be afraid. If you disagree with the bill, fight it before you pay it.*

### Tying It All Together

1. *Know Your Rights—Be Aware of Your Medical Benefits.*
2. *Don't You Just Love a Bargain? Compare Prices for Tests at Hospitals and Medical Facilities.*
3. *Ask the Right Questions.*
4. *Check Options for the Medically Uninsured and Under-insured—Call Your State Department of Insurance.*
5. *Look for Discounts on Your Medication.*
6. *Don't Assume Your Bill Is Correct.*
7. *Check All Your Medical Bills for One Visit and Make Sure You Were Not Overcharged.*
8. *Determine Who is Processing Your Medical Bill.*
9. *Learn How to Decode Your Bill.*
10. *Make Sure the Bill is Within Reasonable and Customary Charges.*
11. *Take Action In Order To Decrease Your Bill.*
12. *Fight It Before You Pay It, and Never Be Afraid!*

### A Medical Insurance Advocate Can Help You Recoup Money You are Owed, and Keep You from Paying What You Don't Owe

*Regardless of how good your health insurance plan is, you are bound to bump up against issues regarding payments for services you thought were covered, overpayments, wrongful billing, and denied medical claims at least once in your life.*

*Many baby boomers are also confronting their aging parents' mounting medical needs, healthcare costs, and navigating the murky waters of Medicare, Medicaid, secondary insurers, and ignored medical bills. Depending on their age, they could also be dealing with these issues for themselves.*

*Working with a medical insurance advocate can relieve a lot of this burden, and provide much-needed support to individuals and families who are fighting with their health insurance carriers or healthcare providers over medical bills and claims—or simply need help wading through, organizing, and prioritizing a growing mountain of them. Even if you are well, as a busy entrepreneur or business owner your mind is on other matters related to your business—not on figuring out if you paid too much, if your coverage is right, or if that denied medical claim has merit.*

### What a Medical Insurance Advocate Does

*Let's face it: when someone is dealing with an illness or recovering from surgery, and those bills start flowing in from multiple physicians, hospitals, and rehab centers, it doesn't take long for the situation to become overwhelming and confusing. Sorting through the explanations of benefits and trying to understand exactly what is covered and what is not—often revealed once those unexpected charges come through—can become a burden very quickly.*

*Insurance advocates act as the expert liaisons between patients and providers. They work with patients regarding their health insurance coverage, medical bills and claims, and can handle all communication and paperwork with the insurance carriers as well as medical facilities or service providers. They are the bridge between patients and health insurance companies,* acting on their clients' behalf to get claims passed, to ensure the highest coverage allowed (depending on the health plan), and to enable patients and their families to rest easy knowing their insurance matters are in expert hands.

Many medical insurance advocates also work with elder law and personal injury attorneys to make sure that all their clients' medical claims are processed and paid correctly.

These experienced professionals sort through and resolve clients' medical bills, lien claims, insurance pre-authorizations, denied medical claims, and medical letters of appeal. They can explain those bewildering explanations of benefits and advocate for patients regarding any insurance issues that require expert or objective attention.

# CHAPTER 10

# NERVOUS SYSTEM

## ELEVEN-SYSTEM MEDICAL ASSESSMENT

**The body can be described as being comprised of eleven systems.** Each system is made up of organs, and each organ is further broken down into many tissues and innumerable cells. Systems are organized groups of structures classified as to performing a particular function, as follows:

- Nervous system
- Respiratory system
- Cardiovascular system
- Lymphatic and immune system
- Gastro-intestinal system
- Endocrine system
- Reproductive system
- Urinary system
- Integumentary system
- Skeletal system
- Muscular system

These systems and their disorders are discussed in this and later chapters, with an emphasis on those conditions likely to result in long-term nursing care at home.

**The nervous system is comprised of the brain, spinal cord, nerves, and sensory organs such as the eyes and ears. Impulses are received due to tactile stimulation from the skin, communications via hormones, nerves, and sensory organs. These messages are transmitted to the brain via the spinal cord, integumentary (skin) system, and blood.** In the brain the impulses are translated into fine or gross motor responses as well as active or reactive actions in response to adverse or pleasurable stimuli. The brain also houses memory, cognition, language and many other sophisticated methods of communication and understanding all by way of nerve impulses.

Some of the various nervous systems conditions and care considerations appear below.

*Cerebrovascular Accidents (CVA),* commonly referred to as "strokes," are common, with 800,000 diagnosed yearly. **They rank fourth as a leading cause of death after heart disease, cancer, and pulmonary diseases.** (Recently, some medical specialists have listed medical errors as the third largest cause.) Loss of neurological function can be sudden or gradual due to a long-term bleeding incident into the brain. **Most strokes result from a blood clot that either originated in the brain (thrombosis) or traveled to the brain (embolus).** Once the clot occludes a brain vessel, the area no longer receives sufficient oxygen, causing a cerebral infarction (tissue death). **Brain hemorrhages are another main cause of strokes** and can occur by a tear in a vessel wall, hypertension, or from an injury. As bleeding continues, pressure is placed on the brain tissues, causing brain tissue damage. **Loss of blood flow to the brain results in injury to various parts of the body, causing neurologic deficits.** The injury may be temporary and resolve over time, or cause long-term or permanent disability. The extent and location of the region of the body that is impaired is solely determined by the area of the brain that was damaged. As all bodily functions are controlled by the brain, the possibilities are endless.

*Care Considerations for Cerebrovascular Accidents:*

1) **Paralysis or decreased function to one side of the body** (hemiplegia), to one or both lower, or to one or both upper extremities can occur. Activity difficulties may also be due to loss of sensation, simple weakness, or changes in muscle tone (being spastic or flaccid). Loss of fine or gross motor skills could be apparent. Depending on the injury, various devices could prove helpful, including canes and wheelchairs, as well as many other occupational therapy aids.

2) **Elimination patterns may be altered** and could encompass voiding and/or defecation. Catheterization, whether intermittent or continual, may be required if bladder retraining is unsuccessful. Bowel evacuation might be accomplished by use of medication, enemas, or laxatives if retraining proves ineffective.

3) **Obtaining the proper amount of nutrients** and fluids could be problematic due to lack of appetite, nausea or vomiting, dysphagia (inability to swallow), loss of sensation in the mouth and throat, medication side effects, or facial paralysis. If insufficient quantities are consumed,

a percutaneous gastric feeding tube could be placed for long-term use. Shorter-term aids include centrally placed venous catheters for total parenteral nutrition (TPN).

4) **Perception and sensory deficits** are often present. These may include vision difficulties such as blurred or double vision (diploia). Partial loss of vision (monocular blindness) or total blindness could also result. Disturbances to taste and smell are reported. Touch and skin sensations are often not discriminated, and loss of feeling (neuropathy) could lead to unknowingly received injuries. Dysphasia (decreased speech capacity) may take the form of difficulty producing speech (expressive), understanding speech (receptive), or both (global). Aphasia is an inability to communicate via speech, but also includes inability to understand writing and signs or pictures.

5) **Cognitive function impairment** includes inability to recognize: faces (prosopagnosia), speech versus not speaking sounds (auditory agnosia), objects (visual agnosia), colors (achromatopsia), and visual objects (visual agnosia) to name a few. Apraxia is the inability to use objects properly when there is no muscle deficit.

6) **Skin care is essential** due to possible incontinence, paralysis, lack of sensation, and inability to ask for assistance.

### Alzheimer's and Dementia

The severity and increasing prevalence of these neurological conditions are evident in these quotes from the Alzheimer's Association's alz.org/facts (our emphasis added):

- *Alzheimer's disease is the only cause of death among the top 10 in America that cannot be prevented, cured, or even slowed.*
- *Today, more than 5 million Americans are living with Alzheimer's disease, including an estimated 200,000 under the age of 65. By 2050, as many as 16 million will have the disease.*
- *You can use the free, online Community Resource Finder to easily locate Alzheimer's and dementia resources, programs, and services in your area. To learn more about this comprehensive resource for people facing Alzheimer's or other dementias, visit alz.org/crf.*
- *The Alzheimer's Association's 24/7 helpline provides reliable information and support to people living with Alzheimer's or other dementias, caregivers, health care professionals, and the public. Call toll-free, anytime, day or night, at 800.272.3900.*
- *Since 1982, the Alzheimer's Association has committed over $340 million to more than 2250 scientific investigations with the goal of identifying novel approaches to diagnosis, treatment and—one day—a cure.*
- *Warning Signs of Alzheimer's (alz.org):*

  - *Memory loss that disrupts daily life.*
  - *Challenges in planning or solving problems.*
  - *Difficulty completing familiar tasks at home, at work, or at leisure.*
  - *Confusion with time or place.*
  - *Trouble understanding visual images and spatial relationships.*
  - *New problems with words in speaking or writing.*
  - *Misplacing things and losing the ability to retrace steps.*

- *Decreased or poor judgment.*
- *Withdrawal from work or social activities.*
- *Changes in mood and personality.*

### *Care Considerations for Alzheimer's and Dementia:*

Gary Joseph LeBlanc (2013) has written a clear and concise little book, *Managing Alzheimer's and Dementia Behaviors: Common Sense Caregiving,* which stresses the following:

**Early warning signs** of Alzheimer's include regular difficulties in recalling: dates, appointments, familiar names, and information given minutes before. Reading and numeracy may suffer markedly, despite a flood of excuses.

**Hospitalization** is disruptive and enhances their confusion.

**Dementia** is a general term for cognitive and memory loss, and Alzheimer's is one of the possible causes.

**Early-onset Alzheimer's** afflicts about a half-million people under the age of 65, and is more heritable than the more prevalent Alzheimer's.

Such patients benefit greatly from the maintenance of routines.

**Early in the progression,** patients can have their thoughts readily redirected. Later, this becomes nearly impossible.

**Approach these patients slowly**, gently, looking to see if they recognize you. Introduce yourself, even to family.

**Be prepared not to be recognized** or only after long delay.

**Go with the flow.** "You cannot move them to your world, you have to move into theirs."

**Be prepared for their hallucinations** and delusions. Exhibiting your frustration will only exacerbate the situation.

**Don't debate, elude**. "I just went out and checked. They must have moved."

**Delusions are false beliefs**.

**Hallucinations are false perceptions**.

**Keep the environment well lit**, for safety and to reduce "sundowning."

**Allow your patient a full-minute delay** in responding to you.

**Communicate face-to-face**, not on the run or at a distance.

**Be alert to pain** versus frustration.

**Avoid combat. Retreat**. Don't take verbal abuse personally.

**Most important** asset of a caregiver: **patience,** patience, patience.

Mr. LeBlanc's little book is a bargain at amazon.com for those dealing with such patients. See also the excellent book by Scallan (2015), outlined in our Appendix 2.

Also highly regarded is the book, *The 36-hour Day: A Family Guide to Caring for People Who have Alzheimer Disease, Related Diseases, and Memory Loss, 5th Edition (2011)*, by Nancy L. Mace and Peter V. Rabins, originally published in 1981. It is available in ebook, paperback, audio book, and hardcover editions.

On a personal note, this afternoon, when I [DWC] came to check on my wife and give her a kiss, she asked, "What's your name?" Yesterday, she told me she loved me. Tomorrow? Recently, as I pushed her in the wheelchair along the path through our park-like setting, she said she would like to live to be 100. I commented that would be 29 more years and asked her if she was enjoying her life, and she replied that she was.

***Epilepsy (aka Seizure Disorder)*** is an **abnormal electrical discharge of brain neurons which may be hypersensitive** and react to unknown chemical or environmental stimuli. Seizures may also occur due to metabolic disorders such as hypoglycemia or hyponatremia (deficits in sugar or salt, respectively), infections such as meningitis, fever, drug and environmental toxins, or trauma. They may be unrelated to any known activities or causes, thereby making it difficult to ascertain origins. Patients may experience brief loss of consciousness and/or whole-body convulsions lasting many minutes.

*Care Considerations for Epilepsy:*

1) **Patient may state he has "aura"** which may signal an attack. Precipitating signs may include pungent smells, nausea, dreamy feelings, and visual disturbances as flashing lights.

2) **Patient my experience fear and shame** during seizures due to lost bodily functions; fear from inability to control or predict seizure.

3) **Due to loss of consciousness,** orient patient, explain slowly.

4) **Anoxia (loss of oxygen)** can occur. During and after seizure, monitor oxygen saturation.

5) **Inspect body for any injuries.**

6) **Lasting safety modifications** may need to be enacted which may include perceived loss of freedom by patient, such as restricted driving. Expect some loss of "self" and independence.

7) **Consider adding padding,** removal of rugs, and improving the availability of suction apparatus.

8) **A medical alert bracelet,** along with wallet medical information, is imperative.

*Parkinson's disease* is a **neurological impairment leading to a slow decline in muscle function.** It leads to progressive muscular rigidity and decrease in movement (akinesia), and involuntary tremors. **Often, initiating ambulation is difficult, and the patient is "stuck" and unable to move.** This is a hallmark of the disease. Once initiated, the patient's gait gains momentum that cannot be easily controlled. Tremors are evident and often appear when the extremity is at rest. There is often a unilateral "pill-rolling" tremor. As the disease progresses, it affects the other muscular systems, such as digestion and elimination. Causes of the disease are unknown. This is a disease that affects purposeful muscles versus involuntary muscle movements.

### *Care Considerations for Parkinson's Disease:*

1) **Tremors are prevalent** but decrease during purposeful movements. Patients should utilize all muscles in both upper and lower extremities.

2) In many instances, **the body is bent forward** to initiate movement because it is difficult to get the body in motion. Time and patience are required to initiate motion.

3) While walking, a potential for fall can easily result, due to the bent body position, inability to alter course quickly, and lack of peripheral vision fields due to forward intent. Once in motion, **patient cannot quickly react** nor avoid obstacles.

4) **Other injuries resulting from lack of movement** include bedsores and urinary tract infections (UTI).

5) **Assess for additional deficits,** including loss of balance, speech difficulties (dysarthia), and problems with eating and swallowing (dysphagia).

6) Obtain evaluation of **level of consciousness.**

7) As this is typically a disease of the muscles and not of the mind, **psycho-social evaluation** is paramount.

*Multiple Sclerosis (MS)* is an **autoimmune disease causing defects in the myelin sheath that insulates the nerves that conduct electrical impulses from the brain and the spinal cord** (the central nervous system). Lack of this myelin insulation (demyelination) is similar to a road under construction: impulses may be slowed greatly or blocked completely rather than traveling at a high speed to get to their destination. MS affects the nerves of the eyes and spinal column primarily, but the deficits are not limited to them. However, nerves of the peripheral nervous system are not involved. Often the disease takes years to diagnose due to the characteristic exacerbations and remissions that the disease presents. Signs and symptoms of exacerbations may be transient or last for long periods and may eventually become chronic. **The resulting disabilities depend on the location and extent of the demyelination, and on what remyelination occurs after an exacerbation.**

## *Care Considerations for Multiple Sclerosis:*

1) **During exacerbations, treatment is supportive**, depending on the location affected. This typically includes bed rest, prevention of pressure ulcers, along with bowel and bladder management.

2) **Monitor ventilation and promote deep breathing** and coughing to eliminate stasis of secretions since respiratory muscle can be affected. Monitor oxygen saturation. Provide incentive spirometer for visual reading of deep breathing. **Be aware for signs and symptoms of pneumonia.**

3) **Muscle weakness, spasms and hyper-reflexia** (over-reaction to stimuli) may occur. Ensure precautions for fall

potential and injuries, difficulties swallowing (dysphagia) and potential for aspiration pneumonia, poor gait (ataxia) and speed.

4) **Patient may experience paralysis:** monoplegia, hemiplegia, or quadriplegia (paralysis to one extremity, one side, or all extremities, respectively). Patient safety and care issues are paramount. Frequently aid in or provide range of motion exercises to keep joints fluid and prevent contractures. Prevent foot drop by utilizing high-top footwear. Utilize aids, such as canes and other rehabilitating equipment, to encourage self-care.

5) **Visual disturbances are frequent.** These can range from peripheral vision loss, to blurred vision, to complete blindness. Assess for vision disturbances prior to ambulation or activities of daily living.

6) **Promote bowel and bladder elimination**, and prevent harm to skin from incontinence by using frequent disposable undergarment changes, skin barrier creams or ointments, frequent turning and positioning.

7) **Reassure patient about loss of function** he is experiencing, but make no guarantee that function will be restored. Remissions often occur with this disease, but such are not necessarily complete.

*Myasthenia Gravis* is an **autoimmune disease that affects the nervous system and exhibits as a periodic, progressive, and extreme weakness of voluntary muscles,** which are the group of muscles which we "choose" to utilize for activities. Primarily affecting muscle of the face, lips, eyes, and the activities of chewing and swallowing (mastication), and speech, this disease can affect any skeletal muscle in the body, including those for ambulation. This disease prohibits the conduction of the nerves to the voluntary (skeletal) muscles, and exacerbations occur during repetitive use of those muscles. A very simplified explanation is that there's no gas left in the tank to make the car (skeletal muscle) run. **It is a disease of exacerbations and remissions; often, symptoms worsen during the day but are improved after resting the affected muscle group.** Extreme muscle fatigue that lessens with rest is one of the hallmarks of this disease. There is no cure, but most patients tend to live relatively normal lives, especially when they know their particular symptoms, recognize them, and are able to provide the rest that is necessary to abate exacerbations.

### Care Considerations for Myasthenia Gravis:

1) As **medications are not effective,** there is no "fix" for this disease. The patient must understand that knowledge of his body will be the main treatment.

2) Knowing outward symptoms by the patient and family may provide signs of over-exerted muscles caused by the blocked and weakened transmission of nerve impulses to the muscles. For example, a **dropping or drooping of the eyelid is often evidence of a potential exacerbation.** Prior to the drooping, the patient may be tilting his head back to see better due to the muscle weakness of the eye because the visual field is lessened by the eyelid interference.

3) **Attention should be paid to breathing and ventilation,**

especially during exacerbations. The respiratory muscles can often be compromised, and this could result in hypoventilation. **Not breathing deeply and fully due to reduced muscle accessibility, both inhalation (breathing in) and exhalation (breathing out), decreases could potentially lead to dangerously decreased oxygen input and carbon dioxide output**. In addition, with prolonged decreases in ventilation, respiratory tract infections could develop, including pneumonia. Assess oxygen saturation; promote use of incentive spirometer to encourage deep breaths and full expansion of lungs, and monitor level of consciousness and awareness.

4) **Promote an environment and personal security** that allow and encourage rest when needed.

5) **Understand that loss of ability** due to continued activity, debilitating muscle fatigue, and the losses associated with "wanting to do" but simply "cannot even consider" lead to loss of self-esteem. Encourage patient to schedule down-time.

*Traumatic Brain Injuries (TBI)* produce a range of disturbances, from short-term and slight trauma resulting in no apparent damage, long-term brain dysfunction leading to life-long impairment, to a vegetative state in the most extreme cases. These are injury-induced conditions which cause neurological damage and do not stem from illness or disease. A variety of accidents can cause TBIs, including sports injuries, playground falls, motor vehicle accidents, lack of oxygen (hypoxia), falling off ladders or down stairs. Recovery from any brain injury varies according to the area of the brain impacted as well as the wellness of the individual and how well the patient reacts to treatment and therapy. Examples of these brain injuries include concussions, skull fractures, and hemorrhages.

### Care Considerations for Traumatic Brain Injuries (TBIs):

1) **Constant assessment is necessary** to determine actual consequences of the injury. Time will indicate acute deficits or chronic conditions.

2) **Areas of the injured brain dictate deficits**, and these may include motor skills (weakness, loss of balance, unsteady gait or ataxia, paraplegia, and quadriplegia), sensory changes (blurred vision, decreased acuity, blindness, loss of taste or smell, hearing difficulties, and tinnitus), behavior changes, bowel and bladder incontinence, dizziness or fainting (syncope), swallowing difficulties (dysphagia), chronic headaches, increased sensations to or loss of awareness of various body parts, increased or decreased reflexes, speech difficulties (expressive aphasia, receptive aphasia, anomia), or breathing difficulties.

3) **Physical and occupational therapy** is often necessary. Rest should be provided between care and therapy to promote maximum effectiveness.

4) **Slow-talking and short-term therapy** can aid in decreasing frustration associated with slow progress of therapy.

5) **Ensure airways are protected** if gag and swallowing reflexes are impaired.

6) **Encourage deep breathing** to promote lung expansion and ventilation.

7) **Avoid coughing, straining or bearing down** which can increase intracranial pressure.

8) **Provide skin care and equipment to decrease risk of pressure ulcers.** Turn and position body frequently. Provide an air mattress to increase circulation and decreases stasis of blood.

9) **Assist with range of motion** exercises to avoid deep venous thrombosis.

*Guillain-Barre' Syndrome* is thought to be an **immune disorder that affects the nervous system.** It is hallmarked by acute and **rapidly progressing loss of peripheral nerve transmissions to muscles due to demyelination. This results in muscle weakness, immobility, and paralysis** beginning in the legs and ascending to the arms, body trunk, and face. Often respiratory muscles are affected which hampers breathing. **The disease process takes three distinct phases:** The "acute phase" begins when the first symptoms develop and continues until no further deterioration or loss of function is noted. This phase may last anywhere from one to three weeks typically. During the next few days to weeks, the "plateau phase" occurs. No further loss of function is noted but there is also no betterment. The last phase, "recovery phase" can last months to years but **recovery is usually complete.** This is the time when remyelination occurs and growth of peripheral nervous tissue takes place.

## *Care Considerations for Guillain-Barre' Syndrome:*

1) As the muscles necessary for **respiration** may be involved, assessment must be ongoing to determine loss of function. While the patient is recovering, provide use of incentive spirometer to promote lung expansion.

2) **Paralysis of any or all extremities** is likely. Provide skin care, turn and position, and inspect skin for any breakdown or presence of any deep venous thrombi (DVT, blood clots); check for swelling, reddening, warmth, suddenly visible veins.

3) **Provide gentle massage** to the extremities. Deep massage is not performed due to the possibility of DVTs.

4) If facial muscles are involved, **provide oral care frequently.** It is possible that eyelids will not close properly and completely. Instill eye drops to lubricate them.

5) During recovery when physical and/or occupation therapy is provided, **ensure rest is given** between sessions to promote maximum benefit.

*Sensory Deficits* can occur with **any disease or injury of the nervous system but are not limited to this system solely.** Sensory functions include hearing, vision, speech, taste, smell, and tactile sensitivity. While some modifications to the environment or use of tools may minimize the deficit, this is not the case with deficiencies in taste and smell.

### Care Consideration for Sensory Deficits:

1) **Hearing Difficulties:** Deafness, whether partial or complete, is not only disease-induced but also results from age, environmental noise, medications and viruses. Hearing aids may help mitigate the problem, but other useful measures include using subtitles on the television, speaking directly to the patient so visualization of the lips is possible, speaking clearly and slowly, and decreasing background noise.

2) **Vision Difficulties:** There are many forms of vision deficits; these include decreased acuity, double vision (diplopia), light sensitivity (photophobia), blurred vision and loss of the visual field. There are few measures that can be taken to decrease this state. Utilization of trained professionals can provide teaching to enhance life. However, dependent on the severity, large print face, recorded books, and bright lighting may prove beneficial to some.

3) **Speech Difficulties:** These could be simply the inability to utter sounds (muteness) or a brain impairment called aphasia, the inability to communicate using speech, writing, or signs. It is almost as if communication is attempted between two people speaking two different and unrelated languages. Aphasia can take the form of not being receptive (lack of understanding of words spoken by others) or expressive (inability to speak in meaningful and proper words). Anomia is the inability to recall names of objects. If the patient has some ability such as reading, communication can be maintained via use of written words or signs. Time

and continued education may be beneficial. Frustration and anxiety are common.

4) **Tactile Sensitivity:** Paresthesia is caused by injury to the nerves. If it often painful and unpleasant, and described as a numbness, stinging, tingling, or burning. While there is little that can be done other than medications, running water over the appendage, wax dips, and massage can decrease the discomfort.

# CHAPTER 11

# RESPIRATORY SYSTEM

**The nasal passages, pharynx, larynx, trachea, main bronchus and bronchial tubes, and lungs make up this system.** All of these organs provide respiration, the exchange of gas, or air, between the environment and the body and the process of making it usable for the body. The end product of inhalation, carbon dioxide, is eliminated by exhaling. Inhaling provides oxygen; it is then exchanged on a cellular level, via the alveoli, and transported to all cells via the blood pumped by the heart. It is the alveoli, the main functioning cellular pieces of the respiratory system, along with the bronchial tubes and organs, which connect the inside of the body to the outside environment—and perform gas exchange providing pulmonary functionality.

A wide variety of illnesses and disorders are accompanied by problems with breathing. Often the need for respiratory intervention and assessment is what distinguishes patients who need skilled nursing care at home from those who do not. Some of the various respiratory systems conditions and care considerations are described below.

***Chronic Obstructive Pulmonary Disease (COPD):*** is a long-term (chronic), debilitating, irreversible, and progressive group of lung diseases that results in **air-flow resistance into and/or out of the lungs,** noted by increased expiration time along with an abnormal decreased elasticity of the lungs further decreasing the air flow. This group of pulmonary diseases includes chronic bronchitis and emphysema. Asthma is also included in this group but will be addressed separately.

**Chronic Bronchitis** is a widespread inflammation and/or infection of the lungs causing narrowing and blockage of the bronchial tubes due to increased mucous, and that is the hallmark of the disease: airflow obstruction due to mucous. While it can be acute, if increased mucous and cough are present over a period of time and occurs over consecutive years, it is classified as chronic bronchitis. It is characterized by airway resistance affecting the smaller "limbs" or tubes of the bronchial tree. It does not directly affect the smallest functioning units of the lungs, the alveoli—rather, it is mucous that blocks the smaller tubes, hampering receipt of oxygen to the cellular level, as well as blocking carbon dioxide exchange. Because the airways are obstructed, oxygen transport to the body via the arterial blood system is reduced. Patients with this condition often show productive (phlegm-producing) cough, cyanosis (blueness) of extremities due to decreased oxygenation, and hypoventilation (breathing in an unusually slow and shallow fashion) due to mucus production that blocks sufficient oxygen into airways.

**Emphysema** is very severe; it causes recurrent damage at the cellular level (the alveoli) rather than affecting the bronchial tubes. It is characterized by permanent and abnormal gaps or spaces between alveoli due to alveolar wall destruction. Without these walls, large air spaces (bullae) result, creating an inability for gas exchange to occur: the gaps are too large to permit efficient transport. Ultimately, pulmonary functioning cannot be achieved. Carbon dioxide cannot be released, and oxygen cannot be consumed and made useful. Airflow obstruction is not from mucous, as is the case with chronic bronchitis, but from cellular tissue damage of the lung. Patients with this condition show long and slow exhalation to get rid of trapped carbon dioxide. They are often described as having "barrel-chests," and they have a tendency to use respiratory and abdominal muscles to force air out of their lungs. These patients tend to hyperventilate (breathe especially deeply and rapidly) because they have trapped carbon dioxide and tend to be hypoxic (low on oxygen).

***Care Considerations for COPD (Chronic Obstructive Pulmonary Disease):***

1) **Muscle fatigue often occurs**, due to trapped carbon dioxide that results in an inability to inhale oxygen. This can result in "air hunger." To treat this condition, promote exhalation and inhalation. Monitor for nasal flaring and use of accessory muscles. Other signs are difficulty speaking and trouble breathing (dyspnea) during exertion or at rest.

2) **Position patient to ease breathing.** Place in "tripod" position, where patient rests forearms on a high table and leans forward to expand chest. When in bed, place head of bed to as upright a position as is tolerable, but ensure patient has ability to expand both diaphragm and abdominal muscles essential for deep breaths.

3) **Monitor respirations** for rapid rate and shallowness,

indicating hyperventilation. Have patient perform pursed lip breathing to expel carbon dioxide: breathe in through nose and exhale very slowly through pursed lips (lips drawn into a kissing position). Avoid fatigue and faintness.

4) **Provide supplemental oxygen** at the medically prescribed level only. Too much oxygen can cause oxygen toxicity and resulting carbon dioxide toxicity. (Oxygen is a drug to be maintained at prescribed levels.)

5) **Monitor vital signs,** such as percentage oxygen saturation, heart rate, and respiration rate. These should be within normal range for your patient.

6) **Monitor for loss of appetite** which could occur if mucous is being ingested and causing nausea.

7) **Promote fluids intake** to decrease mucous thickness (and viscosity) and promote expelling mucous.

8) **Perform chest physiotherapy,** including "cupping" of back to loosen secretions.

9) **Ensure medications are taken as prescribed**; these may include bronchodilators, inhalation therapy, diuretics, antibiotics, or steroids. Compliance with instructions is essential.

10) **Reassure the patient**, who may mourn the difficulty in breathing and feel he can no longer participate in life, becoming hopeless. To prevent the experiencing of a loss of self, encourage interaction with others.

11) **Obtain portable oxygen, if it's needed all the time,** to encourage leaving the home and combat isolation.

12) **Provide assistance with care while promoting self-care** as much as possible.

13) **Do activities in short bouts** to decrease fatigue and allow periods of rest in between them. Learn the signs of weariness and exhaustion.

**Asthma:** is a form of chronic obstructive pulmonary disease (COPD) but is often discussed separately from chronic bronchitis and emphysema because episodic symptoms often result from triggers or environmental stimuli and the patient may be asymptomatic between episodes. Airway obstruction can be caused in three different ways, acting separately or collectively: bronchospasms, mucus secretion, and mucosal edema.

Bronchospasms are the narrowing of the bronchial tubes due to contractions of the muscles, causing coughing and wheezing.

Increased mucus production is the result of inflammatory responses to allergic reactions due to outside allergens, causing the release of histamine (extrinsic reaction) or due to effects of non-allergic causes such as emotions or cold weather (intrinsic reaction).

**The thick over-production of mucus, along with edema** (swelling due to fluid build-up) of the bronchial tube lining further constricts the opening of the bronchial tubes. When the patient inhales, the bronchial lumen (space within the tube) is only partially open. However, due to pressures within the body, the lumen closes when the patient exhales, trapping carbon dioxide, and gas exchange at the alveolar level is impaired. Asthma triggers may include anything that causes an allergic reaction, such as dust, pollen, food allergies, as well as conditions including stress, fatigue, exercise, and temperature changes.

### Care Considerations for Asthma:

1) **Learn the triggers of the asthma attacks** and limit the triggers as much as is possible. While it is difficult to eliminate extrinsic triggers such as cold weather, minimizing contact, using scarves, or entering warm cars may discourage attacks.

2) **Proper use of medications**, whether daily or for attacks, is essential. Bronchodilators help to decrease the bronchial constriction and edema while promoting ventilation. Corticosteroids act similar to bronchodilators but also help to decrease the inflammatory and immune response to the allergen.

3) **During attacks, supplemental oxygen** may be necessary if the patient has difficulty breathing (dyspnea) or shows signs of insufficient oxygen intake with increased respiratory rate and depth. Be sure to use proper amount of oxygen, as too much can be as detrimental as too little. Beware of carbon dioxide air trapping.

4) **Pursue effective relaxation techniques**, which could prove vital during an exacerbation. Imagery, yoga, or focused breathing may help to calm patient and decrease

anxiety and fear during an attack when he is unable to breathe.

5) **Promote fluids**, especially after an attack, to help thin secretions and help expel them.

6) **During an attack, position patient to assist in breathing.** He should sit upright and lean forward to promote chest expansion.

7) Because attacks can be episodic, **fear may be constant,** especially if triggers are unknown or unable to be avoided. Teach and reinforce that medications will assist. As the time the patient has been enduring the disease increases, so will his ability to understand and recognize the early signs of an asthma attack.

*Sleep Apnea:* This is defined as temporary absence of breathing during sleep, absences that may last more than 10 seconds and occur thirty times or more in a seven-hour sleep period. When breathing stops for a prolonged period, oxygenation decreases and carbon dioxide levels increase. Sleep is fragmented, and the patient often wakes many times a night. In the morning, he feels he had unsatisfying sleep, may feel drowsy and fatigued, or suffer a morning headache. It is a common condition, and partners are often the first to observe the situation. There are three distinct types of sleep apnea:

**Obstructive sleep apnea** is caused by an inability to keep the upper airway open (patent); the structures in and around the mouth and pharynx collapse or become obstructed. This is usually accompanied by snoring, as the airways start to close, and snorting, which then opens them up.

**Central sleep apnea** does not have sounds associated with it, because it is not due to obstruction but rather is from lack of nervous system communication. This type of apnea strictly involves the part of the brain center that controls respiration and the respiratory muscles that perform the work of breathing. Proper signals are not sent by the brain and thus not directing the muscles to act. Simply stated, the brain has not told the muscles to breathe for the body. This results in no breathing, no movement of the chest, and no breath sounds. This is further marked by excessive daytime sleepiness, such as falling asleep during meetings or while driving, as the body has been deprived of oxygen during these episodes.

The last type is mixed apnea, the combination of the two types.

*Care Considerations for Sleep Apnea:*

1) **Diagnosis is made in a formal sleep study lab**. Encourage participation. Fear of positive diagnosis or embarrassment may prevent patient from undergoing study.

2) **If apnea is due to obstruction, surgical remedy** may be available. Help patient understand the ramifications of surgery, the potential benefits or curative possibility (whether partial or complete). Learn post-surgical complications and healing actions. Provide honest feedback of results.

3) **Many sleep apnea patients are obese**, causing or increasing the incidents of the apnea. Encourage weight loss. Promote healthy foods, increased non-caloric fluids, and exercise. In addition, changes in some underlying

conditions, such as type-2 diabetes or hypertension may occur. Prior to initiating, discuss with physician.

4) **After confirming diagnosis and weight loss does not remedy the condition, treatment may be obtained using a continuous positive airway pressure (CPAP) machine.** Used at night, this machine, with a device that covers the nose and/or mouth, provides a constant mild stream of air that forces the airway to remain open. Ensure that face apparatus fits properly and comfortably, has ample tubing, is set correctly, and functions optimally.

5) **If patient is using a CPAP machine**, he may be uncomfortable initially. Provide support but do not pressure usage. Encourage use by noting positive benefits such as increased energy in morning and during the day, as well as enhanced mood and disposition due to getting a restful night's sleep.

***Respiratory Treatments and Therapies:*** Effective respiration occurs at the cellular level when carbon dioxide and other wastes are exchanged for oxygen via the blood. For this to happen, inhaled oxygen from the environment proceeds within the lung structure comprised of increasingly smaller tubes (the bronchial tree) to the smallest functional unit in the lungs (the alveolus), where gas exchange takes place and transported via the venous system. If there is an inadequate amount of oxygen available in the blood (hypoxemia), then there will be insufficient oxygen to meet the needs of tissues and cells (hypoxia). Any blockage or obstruction, such as mucus, inflammation or infection, prohibits this from happening, and, therefore, decreases pulmonary function. Forms of treatments and therapies to promote respiration include suctioning, eliminating mucus plugs, lavage, chest percussion, and controlled coughing and positioning.

**Suctioning** is used to eliminate excess secretions from a part of the respiratory system to maintain an open airway. Secretions that could cause obstruction may be thin and watery or thick and tenacious. This will vary dependent on location and underlying disease and ventilation assistance that the patient may have. All types of suctioning require attachment to a suction machine via long tubing.

**Oropharyngeal suctioning** uses a rigid plastic catheter with openings, often called a Yankauer suction catheter, to remove oral secretions. It is inserted into the mouth to remove excess liquid; it is often required for patients who have inefficient gag reflexes and an inability to swallow these secretions. Yankauer suctioning removes saliva and mucus that could enter the lungs. Depending on the awareness of the patient, this suction can be done directly by him, as it is much like handling a toothbrush.

**Nasotracheal suctioning** is used to clear secretions from the trachea and lower airways when a patient cannot do so himself. It requires a sterile technique even though the airway access is obtained from the nose. Secretions can range from as thin as saliva to being much thicker in nature.

**Endotracheal and tracheostomy suctioning** is used when there is a direct access to the lower airways, either by intubation or permanent placement of a tracheostomy tube, respectively. This type of ventilation and suction completely bypasses the respiratory system above the trachea. Strict sterile technique is necessary, and often a closed suction tubing suctioning system is used to promote sterility, as well as not requiring the patient be disconnected from a ventilator.

### Care Considerations for Suctioning:

1) **Sterile technique** is essential for all suctioning, except oropharyngeal, as the area below the pharynx is a sterile area. Patients requiring suctioning usually have compromised pulmonary systems and are at risk for respiratory infections.

2) **Ensure proper technique is used.** Insert catheter into airway until resistance is felt or the patient coughs. Pull back slightly and then apply intermittent suction until the catheter is removed. Never apply suction while inserting the catheter.

3) **Patient should be well oxygenated prior to suctioning,** especially if a closed suction system is not used.

**Mucus Plugs** are merely accumulations of mucus, tissues, cells, and dirt that block or obstruct an airway or tube. Patients with artificial airways are more susceptible, because the tubes can stimulate or cause stasis of secretions. In addition, air bypasses the usual defenses, filtration, and humidification of normal airways. However, replacing equipment, such as an inner cannula, or carrying out lower airway suction, often relieves the obstruction. Removing plugs in patients with natural airways are difficult and requires strong forceful coughing, abdominal thrusts, and suctioning. Regardless of the type of airway, mucus plugs must be removed.

### Care Considerations for Treating Mucus Plugs:

1) **Maintenance of and compliance to scheduled equipment usage** is vital to optimal functioning, filtering, and minimizing buildup of secretions.

2) **Increased hydration and humidification** may assist in keeping mucus from hardening. Use caution to prevent fluid overload.

3) **Suctioning, as prescribed,** eliminates the stasis (pooling) of secretions, which minimizes the formation of a mucus plug.

4) **Lavage may (or may not) help to loosen secretions.** (Strictly follow physician's and/or pulmonologist's guidelines.)

**Lavage** (washing out) is a treatment that is not universally recommended and not definitely a commonplace, accepted practice. During lavage, a small amount of normal saline is instilled to stimulate a cough. Once the fluid is delivered, the patient is suctioned. The thought behind lavage is that instilling a small amount of sterile, normal saline into the bronchial tubes will loosen secretions, thereby making them easier to suction and prevent mucus plugs. However, research has not indicated whether this is true. Some theories suggest that instilling fluid, while loosening secretions, may actually disperse bacteria throughout the lung. Alternatively, more humidification and hydration may relieve the mucous plug condition.

*Care Considerations for Lavage:*

Consult your medical professionals and follow their guidelines. Inquire about humidification and hydration for the patient. Follow recommendations concerning care of the equipment.

**Chest Percussion,** also known as Chest Physiotherapy, is done to loosen and help remove secretions that accumulate in the lungs, especially in the bases. It involves using numerous techniques.

Clapping, or percussion, is performed by thumping the hands, held in a cup-like position, against the patient's back. After clapping, postural drainage is then utilized. To achieve this, the patient's body is tilted so his head is lower than his lungs. This aids in the drainage of secretions due to gravity. If a patient is unable to be tilted, suctioning would then be performed.

*Care Considerations for Chest Percussion:*

1) **When cupping, ensure clapping is not too forceful.** The thumping should be strong but should not cause pain or discomfort. Massaging the back with lotion in an upward motion after cupping also aids in movement of secretion as well as provides comfort after the procedure.

2) **Use caution when placing a patient in a head-first downward angle.** Depending on quality of his oxygen status, the patient may be at risk for dizziness and fainting. The angle of the body does not need to be great for adequate postural drainage.

**Controlled Coughing and Positioning:** Correct positioning helps to keep airways clear by promoting ability to expand chest, breathe deeply, and use muscles. While the patient is sitting, the head of the bed should be at a 45- to 60-degree angle (semi-Fowlers) to a 90-degree angle (high Fowler's position). This enables chest expansion, full use of the diaphragm muscle and other respiratory and abdominal muscles. If the patient is standing, and having difficulty breathing, support his body against a wall. This will provide safety as well as support for his back to promote chest expansion. If the patient is lying in bed on his back (supine position), use two or more pillows or raise the head of the bed to a 30-degree angle to promote deep breathing. This is often a better position for patients who have a large abdominal girth.

Controlled coughing is an exercise and technique to clear secretions and maximize the coughing effort. Coughing that does not expel secretions is not effective, causing additional coughing ultimately leading to discomfort and fatigue. Position the patient in a Fowler's position. Often it is more comfortable for the patient to support his abdomen with a pillow. He then takes two slow, deep breaths in through the nose and exhaled through the mouth. At the third breath, inhale through the nose and hold the breath, count to three, then without inhaling between, cough deeply two or three times pushing the air out of the lungs.

### Care Considerations for Controlled Coughing and Positioning:

1) **Ensure patient safety at times.** If the patient is not mobile, ensure turning and positioning is done every two hours to decrease risk of pressure sores.

2) **Be mindful of patient comfort.** When in discomfort, less

effective breathing is performed and is exhibited by shallow breaths, increased or decreased rate, and ultimately a decrease in oxygen saturation.

3) **Monitor oxygen saturation** to provide actual verification of the effectiveness of the position.

4) **Encourage ingestion of fluids** to thin secretions for ease in their expulsion.

5) **Practice controlled coughing exercises**. Count the repetitions and advise patient on steps to perform technique. Support and encourage practice, even if immediate results are not seen.

6) **Observe for correct use of incentive spirometer.** The goal is to maximize exhalation—not inhalation. Patient should take a deep breath in through the nose, and then exhale though the mouth of the machine to make the device's indicator rise. The higher rise of the indicator demonstrates that a deeper exhalation was accomplished.

# CHAPTER 12

# CARDIOVASCULAR SYSTEM

Some classifications separate this system into two distinct systems: the cardiac system and the vascular system. However, they are so interconnected that they are more frequently studied and assessed at the same time. **The cardiovascular system is comprised of the heart and all vessels within the body, called arteries and veins, to the smallest units, called arterioles and capillaries,** respectively, where oxygen transfer occurs.

**The heart is a two-sided, four-chambered muscular organ.** The left side of the heart pumps the oxygen-rich blood it receives from the lungs to all parts of the body. The right side receives oxygen-depleted blood back from the body and returns it to the lungs where it can be re-oxygenated.

The vessels that distribute oxygenated blood from the left side of the heart are arteries. Veins return deoxygenated blood to the right side of the heart, which sends it to the lungs for oxygen replenishment. This system allows for a constant cycling and replenishing of oxygen to the blood which is vital for cellular life.

Some of the various cardiac and vasculature system conditions and care considerations appear below:

*Heart Disease (also called Cardiovascular Disease):* is a general descriptive term used to indicate **an illness or condition that affects any part of the heart and its normal functioning.** It may include the coronary arteries (the arteries that provide oxygen solely to the heart), the electrical conduction system which effects and regulates the heart rhythm, the valves of the heart chambers which regulate blood flow, or the actual muscle of the heart (myocardium).

**Commonly, heart disease is diagnosed after a heart attack** (myocardial infarction or "MI"), which occurs when blood flow to coronary arteries is blocked. MIs usually result from coronary artery disease (CAD), the most common form of heart disease. Narrowing of the coronary arteries' lumens is caused by a build-up of plaque (atherosclerosis). The narrowing of these vessels decreases blood flow to the heart tissue (myocardium). As the openings, lumens, of the cardiac arteries become blocked, the supply of oxygen to the heart decreases. Ultimately, the heart itself doesn't have sufficient oxygen to continue its function. **Heart attacks (MIs) usually result from these blockages, causing ischemia, injury and death of cardiac muscle.**

**This disease could also include angina,** which often presents as a heart attack with the associated symptoms of burning, crushing pressure, or squeezing tightness. Often these symptoms exacerbate with exertion, emotions, increased food consumption, and cold air, and could be preemptive signs of potential heart attacks.

**Defects of any of the four heart valves** (which act as two-way toggle switches) can also be included in this category. Heart valves regulate the amount of blood flow into and out of the heart. They open and close based upon pressures of the fluid within each heart chamber, as well as working with other anatomical structures. Like any pump, the heart requires intake and output valves that regulate the pressures in the chambers of the heart to direct flow from one chamber to the next Once the pressure on one side is maximized, fluid is released and allowed to enter the next chamber.

**When the valves no longer hold complete seals,** blood can leak in or seep out of the chamber, making it difficult to pump blood effectively and completely. Sometimes, valve malfunctions can be detected during regular medical check-ups, due to the sounds picked up using a stethoscope, **"heart murmurs."** Deficits due to heart valve dysfunction diminish the effectiveness of the heart because blood is not contained and regulated completely, causing a decrease in blood that is pumped to the body.

**Arrhythmias (irregular and abnormal heart beatings** and rhythms), and other cardiac conduction issues may also contribute to heart disease but rarely cause the disease itself. Arrhythmias can result from myocardial infarctions, stress, increased caffeine consumption, and various other factors. Over time, they can cause cardiomyopathy (enlarged heart tissue growth), eventually leading to heart failure.

*Care Considerations for Cardiovascular Disease:*

1) **Weight loss and dietary changes** prove most effective.

Decreasing salt decreases potential water weight retention and edema and possible hypertension, thus lessening stress on the heart. **Weight loss** decreases risk for diabetes, paramount in ensuring small blood vessels can provide oxygenated blood to small capillaries that supply the eyes, feet, heart, *etc.* Extra fluid retention causes exertion by the heart muscle, which increases oxygen demand and increases edema into tissues. **Dietary changes**, such as minimizing fats and cholesterol, as well as eating vegetables, fruits, and whole grains, provide additional benefits beside weight loss. These include the decrease or elimination of the need for anti-cholesterol medication (statins) when dietary cholesterol is decreased. With increased fiber, cholesterol is eliminated in the stool. Decreases of sugar and processed sodium allow decreases in hypertensive medication and improved diabetes management.

2) **Smoking cessation** is key, and various aids are available on the market to assist in this endeavor. Even if full elimination is not achieved, decreasing the daily intake of tobacco products is worthwhile.

3) **Regular exercise and decreasing stress** often work hand-in-hand. **Exercise** increases effort by your heart and blood vessels and directly increases blood flow to all parts of your body, strengthening the heart muscle and increasing oxygenation of the body even during rest. **Exercise** also decreases stress because you increase endorphins, which are "brain hormones" that provide feelings of well-being. With exercise, the signs and symptoms of diabetes and excessive fats or lipids in the blood (hyperlipidemia) can be lessened.

4) **Medication** is often prescribed and may alleviate and postpone the adverse symptoms and progression of the disease. Medications that may be prescribed include **anti-hypertensives** (to decrease high blood pressure), **diuretics** (water pills), **statins** (to decrease cholesterol), **beta blockers** (to regulate heart rate and rhythms), **sub-lingual nitroglycerin** (for angina pain and symptoms), and **aspirin** (to decrease platelet aggregation).

5) In severe cases, **surgical intervention** may be required. This includes **coronary artery bypass graft** (CABG) or percutaneous transluminal **coronary angioplasty** (PTCA) during a cardiac catheterization. **Pacemakers** may be surgically implanted to regulate dysrhythmias

*Heart Failure (also called Congestive Heart Failure):* is a disease that **affects the pumping action of one side of the heart,** the left or right ventricle, such that it no longer meets the body's demand for oxygen. It typically is caused from coronary artery disease or myocardial infarctions that weaken the heart muscle.

**The left ventricle** of the heart pumps oxygenated blood received from the lungs to the entire body, via the arteries. When that side of the heart does not pump effectively, fluid is retained in the left ventricle, backs up and returns to the lungs. Pulmonary dysfunction ultimately resulting in loss of oxygen to the body occurs. With diminished oxygenation and pulmonary conges- tion, **the patient may exhibit shortness of breath, diminished and adventitious lung sounds as fluid is retained in the lungs, activity intolerance, high heart rate (tachycardia) due to in- creased oxygen demand, faintness and light headedness.** Blood oxygen is not available to meet the needs of the individual.

**The right side of the heart** and venous system receives deoxygenated blood back from the body sending it to the lungs for oxygen recovery. **If this side of the heart fails**, because the right ventricle cannot eliminate all the liquid, **systemic edema results**. In this case, fluid cannot be eliminated, so it eventually flows back to where it was received, from the body, **primarily notable by swelling in the extremities.** The patient exhibits edema in the extremities and tissues, **unexplained weight gain, abdominal distention, and bloating in organs such as the liver and spleen.** Fluid is trapped. It cannot be eliminated because the right side of the heart cannot effectively pump the fluid received from body tissues. Right-sided heart failure is often secondary to left-sided heart failure.

### *Care Considerations for Heart Failure:*

1) Patients are usually on **fluid restrictions** to decrease the accumulation of fluid that the heart must pump. Strict attention to fluid volume is required and must be measured. In addition, **low-sodium diets** are also key because excess sodium causes the body to hold water.

2) **Medication** to improve heart function and to aid the body is often prescribed. These include **diuretics (water-pills)** to promote elimination of water via the renal system and **cardiac** drugs to increase the heart's pumping action. Other medications may include potassium supplements, if diuretics are used.

3) Because of **pulmonary congestion**, numerous actions should be taken. **Supplemental oxygenation** may be prescribed due to the patient's shortness of breath and

may be used especially during exertion. **Ambulation and activities** should be increased as much as can be tolerated. Utilize a **pulse oximeter (giving blood oxygen level as well as pulse rate)** to ensure adequate oxygen is obtained. In addition, **coughing and deep breathing exercises** should be practiced to promote full expansion of the lungs. **Listen to lung sounds.** Often fluid backs up into these organs and is heard as "crackles". These sounds are typically heard in the lung bases first. **Position head of bed** to a sitting position to promote oxygenation

4) Due to systemic and portal **congestion,** measures are taken to **decrease problems associated with edema.** Fluid is retained in the lower extremities first, due to gravity. Pedal pulses should be checked to ensure continued blood flow. Likewise, check skin color for pallor, cyanosis, and signs of venous stasis which can lead to skin breakdown. **Elevate legs, perform range of motion exercises, and promote ambulation** as tolerated to promote fluid return.

5) **If fluid accumulates in the organs, anorexia and nausea** may be present. Promote frequent small meals rather than large ones. Ensure fluid restrictions are maintained.

*Peripheral Vascular Disease (PVD)*: is a condition that is caused by partial or complete blood flow blockage, typically occurring in the lower extremities. **It may affect both venous and arterial flow,** causing pain and often evidenced by changes to the skin and decreases in pulses in the feet (pedal pulses). Because blood flow is obstructed by atherosclerosis (plaque buildup), a loss of elasticity of the vein walls (arteriosclerosis), clot formation (deep vein thrombosis), or other disease processes, such as diabetes, for example, there is a decrease in oxygen to the extremities if arterial blood flow is obstructed or stasis of blood when pooling of fluid occurs if venous return is compromised. **This condition often results secondary to hypertension (high blood pressure), stroke, diabetes, and hyperlipidemia (high blood cholesterol).** It is a major cause of **amputation. Pain** is the hallmark of the disease and when the pain occurs identifies the origin of the disease.

**Rest pain** (pain during inactivity) occurs with **arterial insufficiency** because there is a decrease in the pumping of the blood by the arteries to the lower extremities. When the body moves, blood is artificially pumped by activity, thus increasing circulatory flow. Reduced blood flow occurs during rest without the movement that pushes blood to the legs and feet. This leads to decreased oxygen to the tissues which results in pain and potential skin breakdown, because tissues die without sufficient oxygen. Typically it's felt as a burning pain that increases when the legs are elevated, because gravity doesn't aid in the transport of oxygenated blood to these far tissues. Blood flow to the legs increases when the legs are lowered (dependent), and pain decreases because the tissues receive oxygen. This pain has been described as cold and numbing because tissues lack oxygen. Skin is pale when elevated, due to lack of arterial (oxygenated) blood circulation. With gravity and movement, the skin color becomes red, circulation increases, and pain decreases.

**Claudication** (derived from Latin meaning lameness) is a **pain that occurs during activity** and is caused by the inability of the vessels to return venous blood back to the heart. This is the opposite of "resting pain." As activity pumps blood to the extremities, because of the insufficiency of valves in the vein or arteriosclerosis, for example, **the fluid is trapped in the vessels, seeps into the tissues and does not transport back to the heart.** The stasis of the deoxygenated blood and consequential edema causes pain. **As activity increases, so does the pooling of the fluid in the lower extremities. When the legs are elevated, cramping and pain subside.** This is classic for this condition. Skin can become shiny and swollen (extremely edematous); pedal pulses are not able to be felt; skin breakdown can occur rapidly.

**Signs and symptoms are quite similar for both conditions and related to oxygen compromise to the tissues, but they result from different causes. As noted above,** what distinguishes these diseases process is **WHEN** the pain occurs—at rest or during activity. **Both have signs** that include **hair loss in the lower extremities, shiny and taunt skin, cold feet and lack or diminished pedal pulses, feet and ankles that are discolored and duskier that other areas of the leg, thick toenails, potential skin breakdown that quickly leads to gangrene and other infectious processes that may lead to systemic involvement.**

*Care Considerations for Peripheral Vascular Disease (PVD):*

1) **Medication** is often prescribed to promote vasodilatation (to open vessels promoting fluid return) as well as low-dose aspirin to decrease blood clot formation.

2) **Smoking cessation and weight reduction** are pivotal in increasing function. Decreases in smoking readily increase circulatory function as well as decreasing venous vasospasms. Weight loss increases ambulatory efficiency in promoting arterial flow and reducing venous stasis.

3) **Assess pedal pulses, extremity and color changes from toes to legs.** Decreases in circulation can be noted in color changes going from toes to thighs. Check perfusion to lower extremities bilaterally (both left and right) using pulse oximeter. Effects of PVD are not bilateral.

4) **Position changes** are effective to enhance circulation and positional shifts should be completed often to decrease skin breakdown. Elevate legs that exhibit venous claudication. Allow gravity to assist arterial flow by keeping legs low if they are exhibiting resting pain. Avoid sitting crossed legged and the use of knee stockings that decrease blood flow.

5) **Warm** colder tissues with light blankets to promote circulation. Caution should be paramount in using electric or hearted blankets; loss of circulation often decreases feeling. This can lead to burns and tissue damage.

6) **Exercise** promotes circulation. It promotes collateral circulation to establish additional vessels to aid in decreasing edema. If pain develops, rest is necessary to prevent fluid overload. In addition, exercise promotes transport of oxygen and nutrients to the tissues.

7) **Skin and foot care** should be meticulous. Wash and dry without rubbing, which may damage skin. Pay special attention to the areas between the toes. Use lotion and powder as appropriate. Mirrors can be used to examine feet for breakdown, ulcers, and necrotic areas, common with arterial insufficiency or venous stasis. Seek professional help.

**Deep Venous Thrombosis (DVT):** is a condition caused by a clot (thrombus) that is usually lodged in a deep tissue of one of the lower extremities. The clot can result in partial or complete obstruction of the vein's flow. The obstruction's ensuing stasis (stopping of normal flow) of blood can lead to severe edema, loss of pulses and loss of oxygenation below the clot. This can eventually lead to tissue death, necrosis, and amputation if prolonged. However, this is not the major and most life threatening result of a DVT.

**The venous system returns blood from the body back to the heart and eventually to the lungs for reoxygenation.** A thrombosis can dislodge, travel anywhere in the venous system, and then settle in a new place where it again halts blood flow to that tissue. This traveling thrombosis is called an embolus. Emboli may lodge in the heart arteries (causing MIs) or the brain (causing stokes). But more often they terminate in the lungs, termed a pulmonary embolus, causing respiratory failure and potentially death.

**This condition often occurs during a post-operative phase,** due to prolonged sitting and inactivity, and any illness that prohibits blood flow and return to the lower extremities, such as diabetes, right-sided heart failure, and prolonged episodes of bed rest, as well as use of oral contraceptives and estrogen therapy.

*Care Considerations for Deep Venous Thrombosis (DVT):*

1) The goal is to **reduce and eliminate the thrombus** and prevent it from traveling, especially to the lungs. This is achieved by increasing tissue perfusion, minimizing risks, and administration of anti-coagulants.

2) **Check both extremities for skin color, temperature, and edema.** The affected appendage may show pallor (paleness), warmth, and puffiness which may range from mild to severe. Check pulses by applying pulse oximeter to one of the toes on both feet. Perform all tasks to both sides (bilaterally) and note differences (asymmetry) from one side compared to the other. Ideally, without compromise to the venous flow, both sides should be equal.

3) Using a tape measure, **measure and record the circumferences of extremities** at their widest point below the thrombus. Then continue to measure daily. To ensure consistent placement of the tape, initially mark tape position on both extremities to provide accurate placement of the tape measure. This provides a baseline and subsequent gauge of blood flow increases or further obstruction.

4) **Anti-coagulant therapy is often prescribed.** These drugs do not dissolve clots. Rather, they act in preventing additional clot formations as well as maintaining the size of existing clots so they do not increase. These drugs can be taken orally or injected into the tissues. This class of drug is also used for a heart arrhythmia problem called "atrial fibrillation," to help prevent clots from traveling to the brain causing stokes. **These drugs cause decreased coagulation and stop clots from forming. Therefore, they increase risks for bleeding and steps must be taken to minimize these bleeding risks.** Simple steps and tender care are required such as using a soft toothbrush to prevent gum bleeding, shaving with an electric razor to minimize nicks and cuts, refraining from going barefoot,

to decrease feet and toe injuries, wearing gloves to protect hands during home or outside activities, and keeping nasal passages moist with humidification to eliminate dryness and forceful nose blowing. Additionally, contact sports should be excluded, and use of sharp instruments such as cooking or gardening tools must be monitored. **In general, decrease ANY and ALL risks for bleeding while using these drugs. Lastly, avoid any kinds of OTC medications that may potentiate bleeding** which include aspirin, NSAIDS, ibuprofen, Vitamin E, ginko biloba, and any other drug that minimizes blood clot formation.

5) At-home therapies to the affected area may also **increase perfusion to tissues. These include warm compresses,** compression stockings, avoiding crossing one's legs, as continued pressure behind the knees obstructs blood flow. Do not perform rubbing massages to the affected extremity, as this may disrupt and move the blood clot.

6) **Pain is often exhibited.** Administer analgesics, such as Tylenol or other prescribed medication as needed. Due to a swollen and painful appendage, provide pain relief before any physical therapy.

7) It is important to **promote deep breathing** to ensure complete lung expansion. This also assists in utilizing other pulmonary muscles in eliminating fluids. This is especially vital if the patient is on bed rest due to the injury.

8) As appropriate, increase fluid intake. Fluids are necessary to **prevent dehydration.** In addition, lack of fluid

can increase blood thickness (viscosity) and cause additional risk for clots due to blood pooling (venous stasis).

9) Some common **signs of pulmonary distress,** if the DVT dislodges and migrates to the lungs, include impending doom verbalized by the patient (classic sign), trouble breathing (dyspnea) with low pulse oximeter reading, high heart rate (tachycardia), low blood pressure (hypotension), chest pain, and loss of consciousness. **Call 911 immediately!**

# CHAPTER 13

# LYMPHATIC AND IMMUNE SYSTEMS AND CANCER

Again, although these two systems are separate systems, they function together to serve one purpose. The **lymphatic system** is composed of lymphatic fluid (lymph) and the lymph vessels that carry extra proteins, fluids, blood products and cells from the body, returning them to the blood. In addition to the lymph vessels and the fluids which they carry, **lymph organs such as the lymph nodes, lymph nodules, such as tonsils and Peyer's patches in the small intestine, spleen and thymus gland, red bone marrow, as well as the cells (lymphocytes) that provide immunity all function in our immune response.** The lymph organs produce the immune response; the lymph vessels carry the response to the pertinent area.

Although this system is basic in function, it is complex in how it achieves its objectives, which are essential for survival of the body. **It handles three fundamental tasks: 1) to drain excess fluid that is between cells and tissues; 2) to transport fats (lipids) and lipid-soluble vitamins (A, D, E, and K) to the gastrointestinal tract; and perhaps it foremost function, 3) to carry** out immune responses to protect the body from pathogens and invasion.

This section addresses the immune system in general as well as inflammation, infection, and allergies (hypersensivity). But it does not specifically address nursing care at home. Most of the diseases occurring in this system are auto-immune diseases, although some result from an inability to provide an immune response, such as HIV. Medical attention and treatment protocols are handled by medication, diet, life-style changes, monitoring their effectiveness and the body's response to treatment methods. However, if the diseases progress to severe forms, outside intervention such as nursing, occupational and physical therapy may be required. The latter part of this section briefly discusses auto-immune diseases. In addition, other sections of this book address specific auto-immune disorders.

Lymphatic vessels generally run alongside blood vessels. These vessels collect and transport excess fluid (lymph fluid) that is located between cells and tissues (interstitial fluid). In so doing, this system provides a fluid balance for the body. Interstitial fluid is one type of extracellular fluid, a fluid not contained within cells. The other type of extracellular fluid is blood plasma. Lymph fluid, like blood, contains generally the same substances except that lymph lacks red blood cells and large proteins, for example. The lymph fluid is then returned to the cardiovascular system for redistribution by the blood vessels. Also present in the lymph fluid are primary lymphocytes (lymph cells) necessary for immunity.

As fluid is drained and flows from interstitial spaces into lymphatic vessels, these vessels come in contact with many lymph

**nodes** that lie next to these vessels. These lymphatic nodes, often incorrectly called lymph glands, are **responsible for "cleansing" the fluid from bacteria and other dead components.** They are scattered throughout the body but usually reside in clusters in close proximity to each other, such as in the neck, underarm (axilla), and groin (inguinal). **These are the areas that physicians often palpate when someone is ill and they become enlarged with debris related to infection.** These nodes also form lymphocytes, which are a specialized type of white blood cell (leukocyte).

**Lymphatic tissue** is that which **produces lymphocytes to provide protection from foreign invaders. Primary lymph tissue is found in the red bone marrow.** This is present in certain types of "flat" bones such as the breastbone (sternum), the end (epiphysis) of long bones such as the femur, and in the thymus gland. **These are primary tissues because they produce two different types of lymphocytes providing immunity and protection: B-cells and T-cells.** Secondary tissues include the lymph nodes, nodules, and the spleen which produce B-cells only. Most immune responses occur in secondary tissue.

By means of lymphatic vessels and tissues/organs, **this system provides protection by circulating lymphocytes to engage with intruders, destroy them, and eliminate them from the body. This is immunity.** And there are two types of immunity dictated by the lymphatic system: cell-mediated immunity and immunity from antibodies (humoral immunity).

**Immunity Overview:**

The body has a variety of mechanisms that provide general

protection and resistance against invasion even before it requires an immune response. **This first line of defense is called non-specific resistance and it includes the skin, mucous membranes, and body chemicals.** When these barriers are compromised, the body is then susceptible and vulnerable for invasion or disease. The immune responses would then come into play.

**When the skin (epidermis) is intact, it provides a barricade.** It is only when it is damaged by injury, trauma, ingrown hairs, or moisture, for example, that it becomes susceptible to invaders such as bacteria, fungal infections, *etc.* **Mucous membranes** secrete a liquid substance (mucus) that lubricates certain surfaces to prevent them from drying out. In addition, mucus traps substances once they enter the body and aids in their elimination.

**Coughing, sneezing, and nose hairs protect the respiratory system. Saliva** helps to decrease the number of organisms in the mouth and washes the oral surfaces. **Eye blinking** keeps eyes moist so microbes are unable to settle on the surface. **Sweat** from sudoriferous glands not only washes away bacteria on the skin, but contains enzymes that help destroy microorganisms. These enzymes, lysozymes for example, are also found in tears, nasal secretions, saliva, and in gastric fluid. Destroyed bacteria are then engulfed by certain cells in a process called phagocytosis and transported via the lymphatic vessels for elimination from the body.

**An immunity response is extremely specialized,** as it provides the body with a means of protecting itself against specific and distinct invaders. **There are two types of immune responses: cell-mediated** immunity that is dictated by cells, and **antibody-mediated** immunity (humoral immunity) that is directed by antibodies (immunoglobulins). Both are directed against antigens.

**An antigen is the stimulant for an immune response:** an immune response only occurs because an antigen is present. An antigen is the invader that has penetrated the boundaries of the fortress and seeks to overcome the kingdom. These include, for example, bacteria, virus, fungus, foreign invader, microbe, parasites, microorganism, pathogen, *etc.* **In general, an antigen is any substance that is not natural to the body, which has penetrated nonspecific defenses and provokes an immune response.**

*Cell-Mediated Immunity:*

**Cell-mediated immunity (CMI), one response to an antigen, uses one type of lymphocyte, a "T-cell."** While T-cells do not have the ability to recognize foreign bodies themselves, they do leave lymph tissue to pursue foreign entities once called to duty. They rely on another type of white blood cell (leukocyte), a macrophage, to engulf the microbe and mark it for destruction. This is "activation."

**Once the T-cell is activated,** it produces other types of T-cells (helper-T, killer-T, suppressor-T, and memory-T cells). This differentiation allows them to perform varied yet specific roles in the immune response. Each type of T-cell then multiplies by cloning based upon a marker on the foreign body. All of these differentiated and cloned T-cells are identical and carry out specific functions to attack and kill the foreign invader.

**Initially, there is just a small number of T-cells that respond.**

**To reach maximum effect, this first response requires approximately 36 hours.** The exact mechanism of how these T-cells perform their role in this immune response will not be addressed here, however. But, and this is where the specificity of the immune response occurs, the long-lived memory T-cells have the ability to recall the particular antigen that initiated the response. Therefore, **in the future, if the same antigen invades the body, thousands of T-cells will quickly respond.**

**CMI is effective is responding to invaders within cells (intracellular), some cancer cells, and is often negatively involved in the rejection of organ transplants. It also aids in the other type of immune response, antibody-mediated immunity.**

*Antibody-Mediated Immunity:*

**Antibody-mediated immunity (AMI) is similar to CMI in overall function, yet vastly different in how it achieves it.** This type of immune response is also known as a "humoral" response, meaning the immune response comes from the fluid in the body (blood, lymph) rather than intracellularly. This response is exampled by vaccinations and natural exposure to illnesses and disease, and brought about via antibodies. In addition, it also uses prompts and responses from T-cells present in CMI for its initiation.

**A different type of lymphocyte, B-cell,** is used in this response to protect from infection, but more importantly, to protect from reinfection. B-cells do not travel to conquer invaders; they stay and remain in lymph tissue (for example nodes, spleen) until activated by a foreign entity (antigen) and called to action. Some of the B-cells differentiate into plasma cells, while others become memory B-cells. The memory B-cells provide a response to the same invader that is quicker and much more powerful the second time around. Plasma cells, however, secrete a specific antibody that is carried by blood or lymph to the site of the specific invader. AMI is effective against invaders that appear in bodily fluids and those that are outside cells (extracellular) which typically include bacteria.

**Antibodies function in various methods**, and some tasks include neutralizing invaders and blocking toxins so harmful effects are lessened, confining and immobilizing invaders so they are less likely to travel to other parts of the body, causing them to clump together to make phagocytosis and elimination easier, and providing life-long reaction (which may decrease over time, however) to lessen the effects of the same invader after an initial immune response is stimulated.

**There are five categories of antibodies (immunoglobulins, "Ig"):** G, A, M, D, and E. They, however, will not be discussed in depth in this writing. However, some information is necessary. **IgG are the most abundant and generally protect us from bacteria.** This is the only type of antibody that is transferred across the placenta to aid in immunity in newborns. It is the most numerous in the blood providing first response to a pathogen, especially upon reinfection. **IgA** is found in saliva, mucus, and sweat, for example, to provide protection for mucous membranes. **IgM** are the antibodies found in blood ABO groups causing allergic reactions in blood transfusions. **IgD** are primarily used for B-cell activation. **IgE** are typically involved in reactions that involve allergies and hypersensitivity.

*Auto-Immune Diseases:*

As discussed previously, **the immune response is triggered by**

**antigens that are deemed foreign to the body.** Antigens are recognized by certain markers, surface cellular characteristics, which alert the immune response to an invader. However, all cells have markers, including those that belong and are natural to the body. Markers distinguish cells: natural versus foreign. **Normally the body recognizes its own markers and does not attack itself** because these cells belong to the body and are required for survival. This is called self-tolerance. However, **with auto-immune diseases, the body fails to recognize "self" markers** and attacks cells and tissues that belong to the body. B-lymphocytes attack normal cells as if they were responding to invader cells, and because of their capacity for memory and ability to travel via the blood, their effects are often long-lasting.

Consider the U.S. Civil War. The primary distinguishing marker for identification between the North and South on and off the battlefield was the color of their uniforms: blue versus gray, respectively. However, if the color of these uniforms could not be recognized, due to fading, dirt, lack of a coat, whatever the cause, friendly-fire could result and the same side could battle each other rather than the opposition. Loosely speaking, this is what occurs during auto-immune diseases. A failure in self-tolerance causes the immune system to attack itself.

**Auto-immune diseases are quite prevalent.** They involve almost every system in the body and attack numerous tissues. **A brief list includes:** Multiple Sclerosis (MS), Systemic Lupus Erythermatous (SLE), Hemolytic and Pernicious Anemia, Rheumatoid Arthritis (RA), Glomerulonephritis, Insulin-Dependent Diabetes Mellitus (IDDM), Rheumatic Fever, Addition's Disease, Grave's Disease, Myasthenia Gravis, Ulcerative Colitis, Hashimoto's Thyroiditis, as examples. Generally, the treatment for these diseases is medication to suppress the immune system from further attacking these organs. However, it is a fine line because suppressing the immunity leaves the body susceptible for other infections and illnesses.

*Hypersensitivity (Allergic) Reaction & Anaphylaxis:*

**Allergies are associated with stuffy noses, watery eyes, sinus congestion, coughing, rashes or hives *etc.* often due to foods, flora, or medications.** They are caused by overreaction to an antigen (called an "allergen" when associated with allergies). Once the body comes in contact with an allergen, non-specific resistance is initiated. Typically, the first signs of an allergy are diffuse and general. However, upon the second contact, memory cells and possibly antibodies present from the first reaction provide a stronger reaction to the allergen. Some allergy reactions can be simply annoying—however, others can be life-threatening.

**Allergies are immune-mediated responses.** For numerous and often unknown reasons, the body acts negatively towards this allergen and uses specific and non-specific responses to eliminate it. The specific antibody that causes this reaction is IgE. However, cell-mediated responses are often seen, as in reactions with watery eyes and sneezing.

**Common allergens are numerous and encompass many categories; they may be ingested, inhaled, or placed topically on the skin, for example.** They are specific to an individual, and there often appears to be a genetic component involved. Allergens can be food-based, such as peanut butter, milk, eggs, strawberries, and shellfish. **Environmental materials and plants**

that can provoke allergies include dust, ragweed, pollen, mold, poison ivy, and grass. **Medications that trigger allergies include penicillin, ACTH as well as vitamins such as thymine and folic acid.** Vaccines, such as for measles or flu, used to provide an immune response, and composed of a suspension fluid and antigen often cause allergies. But it is often the liquids that carry the vaccine that elicit the allergic response. **Venomous bites** from bees, wasps, and snakes and even topical ointments and cosmetics also can provoke allergies.

**Often, these allergic reactions or irritations are not lethal and merely require avoidance of the substance** (food or drugs) once identified or the use of over-the-counter remedies to lessen symptoms (environmental). However, depending on severity of the response invoked, they can cause a serious, dangerous, and a critical reaction known as anaphylaxis.

**Anaphylaxis is a severe, often life-threatening, reaction to an allergen.** Only one previous exposure to an allergen can initiate this immune response, which may first appear as general and diffuse, with hives or rashes, perhaps some edema around the mouth or wheezing, for example. **Even this first response to the allergen could be very serious, however.** Often, though, is it not until the second exposure when the severity to the allergen is known. The second immune response is severe and quick, and while its function it to protect the body, it often puts the body in danger.

**From inflammatory and immune responses** as well as from the release of other body chemicals, histamines for example, blood vessels dilate so that blood moves faster, often assessed as redness and edema, if the area is external. This, however, causes other structures, such as muscles in the airways to decrease and contract, causing breathing difficulties due to this airway obstruction. As mucus increases, combined with reduced airways, breathing is further compromised. Wheezing and shortness of breath is detected. There can also be decreased cardiovascular functioning caused by the dilation of blood vessels and fluid loss to other parts of the body.

**Severe and systemic anaphylactic reactions require emergency actions to counteract the body's excessive immune response.** This is done by use of an "epi-pen.". This medication, which is administered into the upper thigh via a needle without removing clothes, provides a dose of epinephrine. Epinephrine is the same medication used for cardiac arrests, although in a smaller dosage, to open up the airways and provide support for the cardiac system. Often a second epi-pen injection is required.

### The Inflammatory Process Contrasted with Infection:

There is often a misunderstanding of inflammation versus infection. **Inflammation, dictated by the inflammatory process, is a natural, general, biological, immune response caused by an insult to the body.** This may be a cut, a surgical wound as well as any kind of internal or external tissue trauma.

**Infection** does not have to be present for the body to elicit inflammation. In fact, **inflammation often occurs without infection. However, inflammation is always present when there is infection. Infection happens when bacteria invades that part of the body that was injured.** Inflammation first occurs but if it cannot heal the wound before a pathogen invades it, infection then results.

Inflammation is the response of the body to heal itself. Infection is the invasion of pathogens.

**The inflammatory response** is protective and involves immune cells, blood cells, and other chemical substances. It is an innate, inborn, and a native response because it occurs in reaction to any type of injury in any part of the body and it does not require a particular pathogen or previous history to start the response. Trauma, burns, radiation, bacteria, viruses, temperature extremes, *etc.* can initiate it. **Four classic symptoms of inflammation occur in response to this process: they include redness (rubor), increased warmth (calor), swelling (tumor), and pain (dolor).**

**The inflammatory process** and function is simple and occurs in **three distinct steps after any injury: to eliminate further injury (localization); remove dead cells, damaged tissue, and debris (neutralization); and begin the repair process (resolution).** This is done by increasing blood flow to the area, causing erythema (heat and redness). As the blood flow rushes in, the injury is walled off to protect surrounding tissue. As white blood cells (leukocytes) and other cellular and blood components enter the damaged area, they engulf dead tissue and any bacteria that may be present. Damaged tissue is then replaced by viable functioning cells to promote healing, possibly with the formation of a scar.

The inflammatory response is conservative and general, but It is often modified depending on the nature of the injury, location and site, and the injury's severity. However, sometimes the response is harmful. For example, if the response is insufficient, this can lead to infection and/or increased tissue destruction. If the response is too great, this can lead to hypersensitivity causing hay fever, for example.

**Infection, however, is a trauma to the body that could not be resolved prior to being invaded by bacteria, fungi, or any other pathogen. The presence and growth of these organisms produce tissue damage.** The injury already initiated the inflammatory process. However, if the inflammatory response is insufficient and cannot resolve bacterial infection and growth, infection results.

**Curing infections requires a specific immune response,** a response that is dictated by a specific invader. As white blood cells and other components continue to engulf foreign matter, the wound bed becomes filled with the dead matter of the blood cells and bacteria. This forms pus (purulent exudate). The color of this exudate often is specific to particular bacteria. Particular types of white blood cells are produced and a particular immune response is then initiated: cell-mediated immunity or antibody-mediated immunity, as detailed previously.

The uncontrolled growth of cells within the body, cancer, represents a failure of the immune system, which is why we discuss it here, next.

# CANCER

**The National Center for Chronic Disease and Prevention and Health lists cancer as the second leading cause of deaths in the United States.** It can have a hereditary component, can be environmental; may arise from one single cell that mutates; and unfortunately, often stems from our own unhealthy living. There is no place in the body exempt from cancer. Every bodily system, organ, and cell can be afflicted by cancer. It can affect every one of the eleven systems described herein.

**Cancer is rogue cells that invade healthy tissues with the desire and ability to capture the body. Cancer cells have unique properties that make them more resistant to death and more likely to survive and grow than normal cells.** They grow in the absence of growth factors (autocrine stimulation) and secrete substances to promote blood vessels to grow to them (angiogenesis). Cancer cells overpopulate themselves by lacking contact inhibitors, which usually tell normal cells when viable space is absent. By lacking boundaries, cancer cells migrate to any other part of the body. They wander and are less adhesive to one location, thereby duplicating one tissue's cancer in a completely different tissue (metastasis). Lastly, even with all of these other reproducing abilities, they have a survival mechanism. Normal cells have a self-destructive ability when they are older or damaged (apoptosis). Cancer cells lack apoptosis.

**The specific care for the cancer patient is often unique, depending on the tissue or system that has the cancer.** All those possibilities cannot be addressed here. In addition, methods to treat cancer are also quite varied; **they include chemotherapy, radiation, immunotherapy, surgery, and any combination** of these, depending on the cancer location and stage, and the health of the patient.

In general, we can provide some guidelines here.

### Nutrition

Regardless of the method used to treat cancer, adequate

nutrition by way of proteins and fluids are essential. The patient may be anorexic. Nausea and vomiting are often present. the mouth may be inflamed (stomatitis) and cause pain, preventing ingestion by mouth. The patient may have an inability to taste food, decreasing desire to eat. Gag reflexes could be diminished, making the patient susceptible to aspiration pneumonia.

Some ways to battle these circumstances are listed below. Both natural and medically provided methods to obtain nutrition are noted:

- Small, frequent meals;
- Bland or non-spicy foods;
- Soft foods;
- Frequent mouth care including washes with non-alcohol-containing fluids;
- Protein drinks, electrolyte fluids, non-diuretic drinks; and
- Comfort food—whatever they may want which they can tolerate to enhance natural consumption. Unless discouraged by oncologists and medical professionals, during treatment, nutrition is essential and usually encouraged in any form.
- Central Venous Catheters, such as mediports surgically implanted in the chest wall, provide long-term access to a large vein just above or at the entrance of the heart, necessary for total parenteral nutrition lasting for years and for chemotherapy. Peripherally Inserted Central Catheters (PICC lines), placed in an arm, provide shorter-term access, for about one month. Special nutritional preparations are available for all these accesses besides allowing venous access for chemotherapy.

- Nasogastric Tubes are for short-term use; they require care due to risk for aspiration pneumonia and skin breakdown where the tube rests on the skin. Pumps usually administer feedings on a slow and regular hourly basis throughout the day. A small flexible tube is inserted in the nostril (nares) down into the esophagus and into the stomach to deliver the nutrient. The placement of the tube is non-surgical and eliminates those risks, but can be uncomfortable.
- Percutaneous Endoscopic Gastrostomy (PEG) or Jejunostomy (PEJ) tubes provide for successful long-term use when changed regularly and with proper care. Inserted directly through the skin and abdominal wall into gastric region or small intestine, the tube bypasses the pulmonary system, thereby decreasing risk of aspiration pneumonia, without eliminating it.

## Musculoskeletal and Skin Care

Emphasis should be placed on the patient's skin and on the range of motion. Due to problems of nutrition, medical treatments, and general apathy and weakness, problems to these areas could be numerous and rapid in their presentation.

In general, some guidelines are as follows:

**Provide basic skin care as you would provide to yourself.** The skin should be washed frequently, dried, and lotion applied as needed and as desired. The skin is the largest organ and requires protein for healing and basic metabolic functions to replenish it. In a weakened state, your patient may be lethargic and not do basic turning functions. Without movement, the skin breaks down. If you add perspiration, bodily fluids, and nutritional deficiencies, the potential ramifications could prove deadly. By simply providing basic skin care often, you are accomplishing waste removal, cleansing, and assessment of the overall condition of the skin. This skin assessment, especially if your patient is undergoing radiation treatments, provides early recognition of skin damage. In addition, the warmth of the water, the aroma of the soap and lotion, and the touch on the skin can also be very psychologically therapeutic to your patient.

**Wash your patient's hair**. This doesn't have to be done daily but should be done in some manner. Not only does it provide a loving kindness, the residuals of nightly sweats and odors are eliminated. It may well not be the upmost medical treatment that is provided, but it is one that may lift your patient's mood the most.

**While performing the bath, or at various times throughout the day, provide range-of-motion exercises.** In a weakened state, your patient will not be ambulating as usual. Joints will get stiff, and ultimately the motion range will decrease if the joints are not exercised regularly. Exercise the joints in an orderly motion starting with the largest joints, such as the shoulder, then working to the smallest in progression, for example: to the elbow, wrist, fingers, and finger joints. Encourage the patient to move often and to participate in these exercises. The more the patients can do for themselves, the better their skin will be maintained, as they will be moving, their self-esteem is enhanced, and they may have less damage to these areas, requiring less rehabilitation time.

**Encourage movement, exercise, and ambulation in any form.**

Just a simple walk to and from the kitchen or from the bedroom to the bathroom provides support for the skeletal system. It strengthens muscles, encourages appetite, promotes balance, prohibits foot drop, and all this is accomplished by merely keeping the patient active. Once a patient is bedridden, it is far more difficult to reverse the process.

**Pain Management**

**Cancer often causes a great amount of pain.** Observe if your patient is experiencing any discomfort. Ask the patient to rate the pain on a scale of one to ten, where one is no pain and ten is the worst possible. **Administer pain medication as needed and do not be afraid to advocate for your family member and discuss the situation with their doctor and nurse.** It is important to note that while in severe pain, your patient will be unable to eat, sleep, or perform any activities of daily living.

While the treatments for cancer will vary and the ramifications from the disease process are numerous, dependent on the type, stage, and severity, you can provide these simple remedial measures. They may be simple and obvious, but they can be forgotten while in the midst of managing care for your family member.

# CHAPTER 14

# GASTRO-INTESTINAL (DIGESTIVE) SYSTEM

Incredibly simplified, this system could be described as one large tube that **begins with the consuming of food at the mouth and ends where it is fully processed and eliminated as stool.** When food enters the oral cavity (mouth), digestion is initiated. Food is then processed with saliva and mastication (chewing), flows to the pharynx to the esophagus via swallowing and peristalsis (an involuntary, wavelike muscular movement to propel contents forward), where it eventually arrives at the stomach.

**While in the stomach, muscular action and gastric juices further break down the food into a liquid mass (chyme).** Various substances, such as enzymes from the pancreas, gallbladder, and liver are added as chyme flows to the small intestines, again by peristalsis. In the small intestines (where "small" denotes diameter and not length), nutrients are microscopically absorbed. The non-absorbed material is then propelled via peristalsis to the large intestines or colon (large in diameter but not length compared to the small intestine). The large colon takes out all usable fluid to return it back to the body, and removes what the body cannot utilize, waste, in the form of stool, which is excreted.

Some of the various gastro-intestinal system conditions and care considerations that may be experienced in the home-care setting appear below.

*Colostomy:* is a **surgical procedure** that takes a piece of the large intestine and routes it through the abdominal wall via an opening (stoma) outside the body. Stool is then excreted via the stoma into a containing bag (appliance) outside the body. This bypasses the normal defecation process, which would utilize the entire large colon, rectum, and anus. The farther (distal) part of the removed (resected) colon is closed and becomes non-functional to allow healing to that site. A colostomy can usually be performed at any area of the large colon, to allow elimination of feces when the normal route is suspended due to severe illness, infection, cancer, obstruction, perforation or any similar process that requires the bowel to rest and heal.

**A colostomy may be temporary or permanent, depending on the underlying illness that requires this intervention.** Temporary colostomies are performed to allow healing, for example, when a part of the large intestine has been removed (resected) and requires rest. Once the two ends are appropriately healed, these ends might be reattached to each other (anastomosis), and normal bowel function may be achieved. However, permanent colostomies are necessary at times.

**Depending on the location of the resection**, and with bowel retraining, a new normal elimination pattern can be resumed via the outside appliance, and with it, normal functioning for the patient. If the location of the colostomy is at the descending or sigmoid colon, a bowel training program may be undertaken to evacuate the colon at a routine time. This is called Bowel

Irrigation. Its purpose is to empty the colon of gas, mucus, and feces at daily scheduled times to establish regularity and decrease elimination throughout the day. This is achieved by instilling fluids into the colostomy daily and at a consistent time to prompt evacuation. It is not a guaranteed procedure, but it has often been effective in providing learned evacuation, depending on patient cooperation and reliability. Areas proximal (earlier on in the digestive tract) have decreased bowel training possibilities. **The area of the colon that is affected or resected largely determines the success of bowel training.**

*Care Considerations for Colostomies:*

1) **Bowel function typically resumes 3 to 6 days post-surgery.** The effluent (discharge) will initially be liquid regardless of where the colostomy was placed. Continue with fluids, including water and substances that provide electrolytes, as these will be lost in the effluent and require replacement. Abstain from alcohol, caffeinated beverages, and any liquids that have diuretic actions.

2) **Change in effluent over time is typical** and also dependent on the colostomy site. A major function of the large intestine is to remove water from processed food material and return it to the body. If a colostomy is performed close to the small intestine, effluent will be liquid because the large intestine has had minimal opportunity to recapture water. The farther along in the digestive tract the colostomy is performed, the more water is removed, and the stool becomes more formed. Generally, you can expect that **if the colostomy was performed in the transverse colon**, because water remains in the stool, the

effluent will be soft, mushy and with potential irritation to the stoma if leakage occurs. **If the colostomy is at the descending or sigmoid colon**, effluent will be more solid, since more fluid was extracted by the colon, and less irritating to the stoma, because it is less liquid and irritating.

3) **The stoma requires constant assessment.** The stoma is made from a piece of the large intestine that is repositioned to protrude above the skin surface. The newly formed, surgically made stoma functions to eliminate waste via medical equipment for containment rather than evacuation via the rectum and anus. The stoma should be assessed for irritation, abrasions or trauma (excoriation) from dressings or effluent discharge. The stoma, itself, should be smooth, cherry red, with a slight amount of edema. **Discoloration, excessive edema and discharge, signs of infection, fever, and foul smell may be indications of decreases in stoma viability.** Consult medical professionals.

4) **Because of the surgical manipulation and delicate tissue, this stoma site must receive the utmost care.** Gently cleanse with mild soap and dry thoroughly. Apply the drainage bag and adhesives ring so the fit is close to the stoma and makes a firm seal to prevent leakage of effluent. Watch for constricting the stoma, however. Use skin barriers before applying the drainage bag and cover the skin around the stoma site. **But do not treat the stoma itself with any kind of barrier.** These actions help to create seals, protect surrounding skin, and ensure stoma remains intact, healthy, and functional.

5) **Application of the bag requires time and patience** to assure firm seal and smooth application of drainage pouch. It takes practice. Allow time to master this task.

6) **Bathing requires consideration and preparation.** Tape bag securely in place to protect the stoma. Use mild soap, rinse, and dry thoroughly without rubbing. Change the appliance after bathing. Always protect the skin around the stoma, as well as the stoma itself, by cleansing with a soft cloth and mild soap to remove the adhesives, intestinal enzymes and fecal residual. If the stoma is placed in the upper colon, and once the site is healed, consider placement of a tampon to temporarily contain fecal discharge.

7) **Monitor amount of effluent and discharge contained in the appliance bag.** Consider changing bag when it's approximately 1/3 full or before the weight of the bag causes any separation.

8) **Post-surgical diet will change over time. Initially, eat a low-fiber diet** (includes only cooked skinless vegetables—no salads and nothing raw; canned fruit; juices without fiber; white refined flours, breads and pasta— no nuts, whole grains, or seeds; lean proteins). Add new foods gradually and observe effects. Avoid anything that may cause gas, foul smells.

9) **Assess and note changes in effluent.** Soon after placement, there should be some uniformity and consistency in the stool, dependent on details of the surgical placement of the colostomy. Placement of the colostomy dictates

stool consistency. As noted above, a stoma placed closer to the rectum will form more solid stools and one farther from there will have stools that will be more liquid. **Be aware of changes in stool color and consistency outside of this norm.** Changes can be indications of potential problems with colostomy function or with diet.

10) **Assess patient functional ability, willingness, and commitment to perform treatment.** Motor skills and visual abilities are necessary to provide stoma care and manipulate appliances. Proper skin care technique to the stoma and surrounding tissue is essential. Home situations should lend to privacy, especially if irrigation will be completed. A separate bathroom is ideal, allowing for privacy and unconstrained time, perhaps in excess of one hour uninterrupted time to fully complete bowel irrigation and evacuation.

11) **Monitor and beware of nutrition.** Fluid shifts are common leading to dehydration. Foods, including vitamins and medications, may be processed differently.

12) **Body image and self-esteem are often greatly diminished.** Lack of such a bodily function often leads to fear in social situations, embarrassment, and decreased self-respect due to lack of bodily control. Reassure patient that with understanding, patience, and obtaining a new normal, whether using a temporary or permanent colostomy, life is usually impacted much less than is initially anticipated.

*Dysphagia:* is a term indicating **difficulty or inability to swallow.**

The act of swallowing requires use of nerves as well as voluntary and involuntary muscles associated with the jaw, tongue, pharynx, and esophagus. Dysphagia can occur for numerous reasons and is often limited to affecting either the esophagus or the pharynx. **Esophageal dysphagia affects involuntary muscles** and can be caused by spasms, narrowing of the esophagus (esophageal strictures) which greatly slows forward progression of food, tumors, and achalasia, in which the sphincter between the esophagus and stomach doesn't relax, resulting in actual trapping of food in the lower esophagus. **Pharyngeal dysphagia often affects voluntary muscles**, which may be damaged by neurological disorders, such as Parkinson's disease, multiple sclerosis, muscular dystrophy, or damage from strokes, traumatic brain injuries, and spinal cord injuries. Complications of dysphagia include malnutrition, weight loss, and dehydration. However, often respiratory complications result when food enters the pulmonary system via the trachea instead of the esophagus. **Aspiration pneumonia and respiratory infections often result.**

*Care Considerations for Dysphagia:*

1) **Evaluate ability to swallow effectively prior to eating each meal.** Check for drooling, speech problems, and patient willingness. Lack of oral control can be an indicator for aspiration potential. Verify patient ability to cough on command. If aspiration should occur, the gag reflex and coughing are essential to decrease aspiration.

2) **Food placement and patient positioning is often critical to enhance swallowing effectiveness.** Sit patient in upright position to increase effect of gravity, as well as have patient tip head back when chewing and swallowing. If

dysphagia is due to a neurological deficiency, then place food on the unaffected side of the mouth to enhance chewing ability.

3) **Mealtime often becomes a chore for patients with dysphagia**. The work required to eat, as well as changes to diet, frequently eliminates satisfaction and enjoyment of this social time. Suggest a swallowing technique that includes gently placing the patient's hand on the throat to feel the action of swallowing. Feeling the motion often leads to enhanced swallowing effort. Additionally, sometimes swallowing two times in quick succession proves effective. Decrease noise and distractions to enhance the effort and concentration of eating. Provide coaching and verbal step-by-step reminders for patients with neurological deficits. This might include: open mouth; feel food in your mouth; chew food until the food is soft without big pieces; tilt head up; swallow; swallow again, *etc.*

4) **Food texture plays an important role with dysphagia.** Liquids are often not given, as they are difficult to control in the mouth, and along with solids, liquids pose the most aspiration threat. Often, the best consistency is that of mashed potatoes, which can be controlled in the mouth and allow some chewing, but can also slide down the throat. This is considered a puree diet which can be further categorized into thin, thick, pre-mashed, or fork-mashed puree. The diet selected by the physician will be dependent on the patient's willingness and ability.

5) **Severe cases of dysphagia may require procedures to widen the esophagus,** for example, or placement of a feeding tube when swallowing food or liquids poses a threat to patient's safety, and/or when malnutrition and fluid deficits are advanced. If a feeding tube is utilized, ensure that the patient's liquid diet is well balanced and provides all nutritional requirements. Numerous types and selections are available. **Keep records of all feedings, water, and liquids that are given to the patient to ensure satiety, caloric intake, and hydration.** Monitor and clean the feeding tube site as recommended by the physician. Be alert to leakage of stomach contents and acids which are caustic to the skin. Obtaining patient weight at frequent intervals is often recommended to ensure too much weight isn't lost or gained.

6) **Understand that eating provides not only nutritional benefits, but also social time and personal pleasures**. There are losses associated with drastic diet changes. The act of eating and chewing provides an individual release and satiety that is often associated with shared personal experiences. With dysphagia, food consistencies are usually altered to soft foods, often discouraging the eating of favorite foods or eating from menu items. Eating pleasures are initially considered restricted. Understand that while these meal-time limitations may initially decrease eating pleasure, social and basic satisfaction of the shared meal need not be denied.

*Altered Bowel Elimination:* **elimination is simply the removal (defecation) of waste products from the body via the large intestine.** The end product of defecation is stool. This is achieved by the coordinated efforts of involuntary and voluntary muscular movements of the digestive system, starting with eating and ending with defecating. Involuntary muscles, of which the individual has no control, contract and relax to push contents (either food or stool) forward by muscular action (peristalsis). Voluntary muscles, controlled by the individual, allow for self-determined relaxation and contraction of sphincters to finally release stool via the anus. Individual elimination of stool varies and may occur once per day, a few times daily, or once every other day. What matters most is that an individual has consistent bowel movements that are neither hard and require straining to expel, nor loose or watery stool. Incidences of constipation or liquid bowel movements should be addressed with a physician.

Often patients with ongoing care are prone to bowel irregularities which may affect the quantity and/or quality of their stool. Reasons for this include multiple medications which can cause various gastrointestinal side-effects, restricted mobility due to illness or injury, changes in eating habits or nutrition or cognition impairments. This can range from constipation to diarrhea, both of which are at opposite ends of the normal bowel elimination spectrum.

### Care Considerations for Constipation:

1) **It is often not easy to ascertain the cause of constipation,** which is a decrease in regularity, difficult passage of hard, dry stool, and often with incomplete elimination of feces. Determining the cause not only helps to select the best treatment option, it also aids in eliminating ongoing constipation patterns.

2) **Medications often cause constipation.** Pain-relieving drugs, such as opiates, so frequently cause constipation that it's common that a mild stool softener or laxative is suggested when these drugs are prescribed. Anti-depressants and some cardiac drugs can also effect bowel elimination. Because these medications are usually prescribed long-term, artificial measures to resolve constipation should be as minimal as possible due to the potential negative long-term effects of laxative use.

3) **Some disease processes can contribute to constipation**. Hypothyroidism or other metabolic disorders can decrease functionality of the bowels. A chronic heart failure patient often has fluid intake restrictions which could lead to hard stools that are difficult to pass. Patients may exhibit gastrointestinal uniqueness such as slow transit constipation (a process in which peristalsis is slower than normal), have a longer than usual colon with overlapping segments (redundant colon) or may have a colon that anatomically twists and turns more than usual making stool passage difficult. Ensure constipation issues are discussed with the physician and follow appropriate guidelines.

4) **Constipation due to lack of fiber can easily be resolved.** Dietary fiber adds bulk to stool to aid passage through the large intestine because bulk doesn't fully digest. Most plant foods have both soluble and insoluble fiber. An additional benefit of insoluble fiber is that stool also retains some water, which helps to keep stool soft for easier passage. However, fiber can also be added to a diet by using over-the-counter fiber supplements, such

as Citrucel or Metamucil for example. These capsules, or powders added to fluid, taken daily can increase fiber intake. Supplements are often used for a patient who is unable to eat or for individuals that can't or won't increase dietary fiber due to the increase of food that is required or from distaste of food that provides it.

5) **A major function of the large intestine is to retrieve and return fluid from waste back to the body for use.** When there is insufficient fluid intake, more water is removed from waste. Feces then become harder, more difficult, and perhaps more painful to pass. This all leads to increased risk for constipation. Fluid should be drunk often. There is no standard amount to drink, but **a rule of thumb is that when one feels thirsty, one is already exhibiting signs of fluid dehydration.** Decrease caffeinated beverages such as coffee, tea, and cola. Juices increase fluids but also increase sugar. Water is often the preferred beverage to consume.

6) **Sedentary lifestyle, often the case for a home-care patient, contributes greatly to constipation.** The elimination of feces is largely controlled by involuntary muscular movements. When the body remains at rest, the body minimizes metabolism, peristalsis decreases, and bodily functions revert to a lower level of expenditure and usage. Simple movement, such as walking, promotes increased involuntary muscular functions, as well as all the additional health benefits associated with exercise. In addition, when one is sedentary, food consumption that maintained a normal weight may now be more caloric than is necessary. A sedentary patient may

also experience boredom. Often, eating resolves that emotional feeling. Unfortunately, the snacks desired are usually those that do not provide increased fiber to the diet. For a bed-ridden patient, range-of-motion exercises decrease sustained loss of muscle mass. Decreasing the amount of caloric intake, as well as increasing fluids, should be considered.

7) **Various types of over-the-counter laxatives are available to help resolve constipation**. However, they may have side effects such as bloating, gas, or cramping for example. Stool softeners, such as Colace (docusate sodium) or Miralax (glycolax), increase water in the bowels. With the additional water, stools pass more easily and without a great amount of strain. The additional fluid also helps to promote and stimulate bowel movements. These medications do not damage the normal action of the colon and are not addicting. Other laxatives, such as Senokot (senna) and Dulcolax actually enhance the action of the large intestine to increase forward movement and release of stool. This works to promote the large intestine's normal function. Because this is artificially increasing the colon's peristalsis, long-term use could be detrimental. Therefore, these, and any other laxative assisting medications should be used as infrequently as possible. Another type of laxative is to be used infrequently and with physician consult: saline laxatives take fluid from the body, due to their composition, and return it to the colon. However, with the fluid, essential electrolytes necessary for cardiac function, for example, are also removed. These laxatives are often prescribed as bowel prep for testing and procedures, such as a

colonoscopy when the colon needs to be free and clean of all feces. **Before administering, consult with the patient's physician.**

8) **Digital disimpaction may be necessary at times when previous methods to resolve constipation are ineffective.** This procedure is often both embarrassing and uncomfortable to the patient. It also has adverse complications, such as vagal nerve stimulation, which decreases heart rate. Additionally, the digital irritation can cause bleeding as well as discomfort in passing stool. A gloved hand with a lubricated finger is inserted into the anus to gently but firmly remove stool from the rectum. Often that will stimulate a bowel movement. If it doesn't, stool removal may provide some relief for the patient.

9) **Enemas, inserted into the anus to provide lubrication up to the rectum, are used break up stool for elimination.** They are used **as a last effort to relieve constipation**, partially due to the discomfort and embarrassment they may cause to the patient. However, they are also detrimental to the body as they disrupt the normal bodily process and cause dependence. Frequent use of enemas causes shut-down of effort, and just a few usages sometimes decreases the body's ability to normally expel feces. **Enemas should only be used when all other interventions fail to evacuate the patient's bowel.** For an enema using small amount of fluid, place the patient on the left side with right leg over the left for support and both knees flexed to chest. Ensure towels, bedpan, and cleaning items are readily available. Have the patient breathe out though the mouth, which helps to relax

the external sphincter. Assess for hemorrhoids that could decrease visual ability for placing the enema tube and/or increase risk for bleeding. Lubricate tip of enema tube, separate buttocks, and insert tip of enema tube into the anus to instill fluid. The fluid should be retained for a period as indicated per package or physician instructions for best results. When the process is complete according to directions, provide full and gentle hygiene to the genitourinary and anal areas. **Be aware that embarrassment and apprehension may be more paramount than the actual discomfort of the process.** Provide gentle care and explain procedural details throughout the process.

### Care Considerations for Diarrhea:

1) **Diarrhea is the presence of unformed stools that may be loose to watery** that occur frequently and are unusual for the patient. Besides the loss of water that is unable to be recaptured normally by the large intestine, essential electrolytes are lost. Ultimately, the patient may exhibit dehydration, heart arrhythmias when the condition is long-lasting, and skin breakdown from recurrent presence and cleaning of stool. This condition can be caused, for example, by diet, infection, food consumption, or medications.

2) **Cause needs to be determined.** Due to the rapid passing of the stools through the large colon, there is insufficient time for the colon to return water from stools back to the body. When water is not recovered by the colon, other essential chemicals, such as electrolytes which aid in cardiac function, are also lost. Look for dietary changes,

gastrointestinal infections, additions of medications such as antibiotics, and changes due to traveling.

3) **Diarrhea may be caused by recent administration of antibiotics which destroy the normal flora of the GI tract.** Often administration of yogurt or other over-the-counter probiotics will help remedy this cause.

4) **Dehydration is often exhibited.** Headaches, decreases in consciousness, decreases in urinary output, and hyperventilation (increased rate of breathing) often occur. Fluid intake needs to offset the fluid lost due to diarrhea. Consult physician should any of these be noted.

5) **Assess the stool for consistency, color, and volume.** This should also be reported to the physician.

6) **Skin breakdown is common with diarrhea.** Check the outer skin for any signs of breakdown such as non-blanchable skin, lack of normal skin tension, or discoloration. Separate the buttocks to view the anus and inner-lying areas for excoriation, abrasions, redness, irritation, or breakdown. Wash and dry gently in a patting motion—do not rub. Apply protective ointments such as A+D Ointment.

7) **Anti-diarrheal medications can be given but caution should be used to ensure their administration does not cause constipation.** Home and over-the-counter remedies include strong tea, rice, whey, Pepto-Bismol. When bouts of diarrhea have decreased, resume the normal diet slowly to further calm and allow healing of the irritated intestinal mucosa (lining) until fully healed.

# CHAPTER 15

# ENDOCRINE SYSTEM AND DIABETES

Working in conjunction with the nervous system, the endocrine system **is responsible for secreting substances, hormones, which are then transported via the circulatory system to target organs. It is the hormones which regulate the proper functioning of the target organs.**

**The secreted hormones regulate numerous bodily processes** and functions such as metabolism, growth and development, tissue function such as insulin release, urinary elimination, reproductive activity, steroid production, and water metabolism for example. The glands which are associated with this system include the pituitary, thyroid, parathyroid, pineal, adrenal, as well as the pancreas, ovaries, and testes which perform other functions as well as endocrine.

**You can liken this system to a home's thermostat which regulates temperature.** If the temperature is too cold, the thermostat turns the heat turn on; upon reaching the desired temperature, or if too hot, the thermostat turns the heat off. The endocrine system works in a similar manner. It ensures that the body maintains an ideal functioning level based upon hormone levels in the blood that are sent to the brain (the thermostat) for evaluation. If the hormonal levels are not optimal, the brain sends signals, via the pituitary, to other endocrine glands which direct target organs to carry out a task. All of this is done via hormones, chemical messages, which turn a target organ on or off.

A portion of the brain, the hypothalamus, by constantly assessing hormone levels in the blood, dictates a gland's release of hormones to maintain optimal body functioning. It is continuous, and **changes are made constantly depending on what the body's needs may be at any given moment.** This is a feedback mechanism, but it is not immediate in its response. The target organ's response time is usually not immediate and prolonged because the hormonal message is delivered via the circulatory system (blood).

As stated previously, hormone levels in the blood are first evaluated in the brain by the hypothalamus. The hypothalamus then sends signals to the pituitary gland. **The pituitary gland, often called the "master gland of the body" causes hormonal release or suppression by any of the endocrine glands.** The target organs then respond so the body maintains an optimal level of function (homeostasis).

Because there are many players in this system, **breakdowns can occur anywhere during this feedback cycle.** This includes: 1) a malfunction occurs between the hypothalamus and pituitary gland; 2) the pituitary gland is unsuccessful in communicating commands to a target gland; 3) the target gland receives instructions from the pituitary but is unable to act on them because it is unable to secrete, or restrain from secreting its hormone; and 4) the target organ of the hormone is unresponsive to the hormone.

**In order to identify a disease process,** it is necessary to determine whether it is a problem of communication between the pituitary and target organ, or simply an inability for the target organ to comply with pituitary's direction to secrete a hormone (hypo-responsiveness).

**Disorders and illnesses from this system result** when a gland secretes too little of a hormone (hypo-secretion), resulting in a hormonal deficiency so homeostasis cannot be maintained. The opposite is also true. If there is an overproduction (hyper-secretion), too much of the hormone is released into the body. **Hormone levels, whether too high or low, create numerous diseases that may require life-long treatment to maintain normal levels.**

**Once the cause of the disorder is determined** based upon specific testing of the pituitary and target gland, the diagnosis typically is handled by medication or surgical removal (excision) of part or all of a gland, but usually one that does not require long-term nursing services. However, diabetes may not be treated this way. Therefore, the focus of this section will be devoted to Diabetes Mellitus.

**Diabetes Mellitus** is a **chronic disease of the endocrine section of the pancreas which secretes insulin. Lack of insulin causes high and damaging levels of sugar in the blood (hyperglycemia).** As a disorder of carbohydrate metabolism, it is evidenced by the body's inability to use nutrients for fuel and storage. This hyperglycemia is the disease's hallmark and is **caused by an inadequate or complete lack of insulin production or resistance to insulin's action.** Other typical signs of the disease include increase urination (polyuria), increased thirst (polydipsia), and increased hunger (polyphagia).

Diabetes is the most common of all endocrine disorders. While the actual cause is not known, there is an auto-immune factor, a life-style and age component, as well as a genetic predisposition. Two types of diabetes are diagnosed and depend on the circumstances and age upon which the disease presents. Regardless, **this is a life-long chronic and incurable disease.** Patients are usually tasked with life-style changes and medication administration to counteract the disease process. **However, with compliance and adherence to proper therapy, in accordance to the patient's underlying health, there can be decreased complications and prolonged life.**

**Under normal functioning, the pancreas secretes insulin into the blood.** The purpose of insulin is to decrease blood glucose (sugar) levels by "transporting" it into cells where it is used as an energy source for normal cellular body functioning as well as to store remaining sugar in the liver in the form of glycogen. This prevents accumulation of sugar in the blood, as it is either stored until it is needed or used for cellular function.

**Without glucose as an energy source, because insulin is not available, the body breaks down fatty acids.** Although short-term energy is provided by fats, their incomplete metabolism creates ketones. **When these ketones accumulate they can cause lasting detrimental effects and death because they lower the pH of the blood (ketoacidosis), which has small range for the body to function.**

**In addition, as fats break down and high levels of sugar remain in the body, blood vessel damage occurs.** Results include atherosclerosis and other cardio-vascular insufficiencies, stroke, nerve damage, peripheral vascular disease and poor circulation, resulting in neuropathy with pain and numbness in extremities, especially feet, along with renal insufficiency and loss requiring dialysis, as well as vision damage or blindness, and skin ulcerations, slow wound healing with associated decreased infection resistance due to decreased blood flow, gangrene, perhaps even amputation.

**Without diabetes, insulin secretion is increased by the pancreas** when **blood glucose levels** rise approximately thirty to sixty minutes after meals to transport glucose for energy. **Insulin levels** then decrease and return to normal two to three hours after glucose levels in the blood decrease.

**With diabetes, without insulin, glucose is not removed from the blood and used for energy,** and the body is required to perform metabolism of other nutrients to obtain energy. To control diabetes, medication (insulin or oral drugs) is given to try to mimic the normal functioning of the pancreas.

**There are two types of diabetes mellitus** which are differentiated by age of onset, etiology (cause) of the disease, and other presenting factors:

**Type 1—IDDM (insulin-dependent diabetes mellitus)** usually presents at 25 years old or less. Its onset is abrupt, and the patient's weight is less than or within the normal range. In fact, the patient may be losing weight even though presenting with polyphagia (increased appetite). **Outstanding is the lack of insulin present.** The reason for this lack may be immune-related, due to genetic predisposition, or of a completely unknown cause (idiopathic). The speed that the pancreas function is destroyed is variable, but the rate happens more rapidly in the young.

**To control this type of diabetes insulin is administered by injection and diet is regulated.** Insulin administration and dosage is very individualized and patient-specific. The goal of insulin injections is to provide the body with a proper level of glucose in the blood for the body to function normally while keeping the levels from becoming dangerously low (hypoglycemia). Often, different types of insulin must be injected to mimic the natural effect of those released by the body, such as rapid, intermediate, and long-acting insulin. In addition, the timing of the injections will vary based upon issues such as the amount of blood glucose that was tested from a blood sample, timing of meals, length and type of exercise performed, the injection site, and the type of insulin that will be injected.

**Levels of glucose in the blood must be tested daily to manage this disease.** By using a drop or two of blood from a finger stick put on a special testing paper, the amount of sugar in the blood is read by machine. This process may occur many times a day. The amount of insulin dictated by a physician (endocrinologist) is then injected into the body. Specific body sites are used to inject insulin because it must be introduced into the skin, not muscle. In addition, different sites use (metabolize) the insulin faster than others, providing more rapid absorption rates, therefore altering peak action times. The sites used for injection include the abdomen, upper arms, thighs, and hips.

**Usually, vascular and neurologic changes eventually develop.** Because the body itself secretes no insulin, and as it is injected into tissues rather than being released as needed, blood glucose levels often fluctuate and are difficult to control within a desired range. **But if detected early, with patient compliance, the manifestations of the disease, although eventually presenting,**

can be offset with proper diet, patient compliance, and medical attention

**Type 2—NIDDM (non-insulin-dependent diabetes mellitus)** occurs more frequently, usually presents after age 40, and is a gradual process. The patient is often obese. Some insulin may be present in the body, but the amount being secreted may be insufficient to meet the body's needs. However, at times there is also a complete deficiency of insulin production. **There is a strong inherited and predisposition to this type of diabetes, but it often lacks auto-immune destruction of the pancreas that typifies Type 1.** These patients do not usually have increased appetites or exhibit weight loss but do suffer from side effects such as itchy skin (pruritus) and numbness (peripheral neuropathy) related to long-lasting glucose and fat metabolism.

**While diet is essential to manage this type of diabetes, medications are often varied.** If the patient is not obese, sometimes dietary changes alone can control it. Oral medications (hypoglycemic medications) may treat the mild/moderate forms of the disease that is usually associated with obesity but not severe enough to require insulin. **There are numerous oral medications, and they work differently on the body.** For example, some may stimulate the pancreas to produce more insulin. Other drugs may work to delay absorption of glucose by acting on digestion by the small intestine. However, **if the patient's glucose levels are not lowered sufficiently using the oral medications, and the disease is severe, insulin may need to be injected.** A variety of medications are tried first to provide a controlled level of sugar in the blood, as determined by finger sticks, prior to initiating injectable medications.

**Compared with Type 1, the same vascular and neurologic changes usually develop.** However, one major difference is that this type of diabetes is usually easy to control and fairly stable once proper medication is determined and the patient is compliant with treatment. But it is important to note that because this diabetes type is long in progressing, it is often diagnosed late, once other complications have manifested.

### Care Considerations for Diabetes Mellitus

1) **Although family members can support the patient, ultimately the patient must have conviction and be self-motivated to comply with the management of diabetes due to life-style changes and blood monitoring, diet restrictions and potentially painful interventions. Medication administration,** especially insulin injections, requires a strict control to maintain blood glucose levels at an optimum range. This may require self-testing of blood before meals, at various times during the day, and before bed. Based upon the blood results, self-administration of insulin, which is injected into the skin, may be required. In addition, **dietary changes** are usually essential. This may include reduction or elimination of favorite foods and/or addition of items that are not preferred. **Life-style modifications**, compliance, and motivation to make these changes are essential for treatment. The patient is responsible for reducing the disease process, or the rapidity of its harmful effects. **The patient must restrict his diet. The patient must test his blood sugar. The patient may possibly inject himself with insulin.** While family members can assist, especially with household dietary changes, ultimately the patient must comply with

a diabetes-friendly diet. Emotional support proves vital, along with support groups and counseling.

2) **Teaching is essential** for the patient to understand the ramifications of diabetes. Compliance is increased when the patient understands the broadly encompassing effects of the disease and damage to vessels which provide oxygen to various structures: eyes, kidneys, skin, for example. **Diabetes can cause secondary problems such as blindness, renal failure which may require dialysis, and osteomyelitis and amputation due to infection, respectively.** A patient's more diligent and active treatment observance to control diabetes, once consequences are detailed, often occurs when complications and progression of the disease are understood.

3) **Finger-sticks are necessary to obtain scientific and measurable levels of glucose in the blood.** Required for insulin injections, these self-tests are also often necessary to determine efficacy of oral hypoglycemic agents. The number of times to test will be dictated by a physician. Initially, and if compliance is a factor, this may need to be performed numerous times a day. **A meaningful record should be maintained not only to capture data but to ensure completion.** Technique in performing finger sticks should be taught by a diabetes-specialist nurse or other professional and the instruction should include at least one family member. A professional in the field will teach the optimum technique. In addition, in times of hypo- or hyperglycemic crisis, someone else can perform testing if the patient is unable to do so.

4) **Management of insulin is required.** Most injectable in-sulins require refrigeration but should be at room tem-perature prior to administration. The patient should verify these requirements with a health-care professional and/ or pharmacist. Improper storage can degrade efficacy of insulin and greatly reduce its effectiveness.

5) **If injecting insulin**, sites of injection matter greatly. Learn and identify the proper sites on the body for administra-tion, which usually include the abdomen, upper arms, thighs, and hips. Each site differs in rate of absorption, and of those listed previously, the abdomen has the most rapid action and the least rapid action is from injections at the hips. Physical constraints may dictate not using a particular site. Sites will likely need to be rotated. Con-sult a medical professional.

6) **When injecting insulin, specialized equipment is essen-tial.** Used often are disposable single-use syringes with attached small 25- or 26- gauge needles that are half-inch in length. These small needles ensure the insulin is delivered into the skin and not the muscle. The small di-ameter of the needle reduces discomfort. (The larger the gauge of the needle indicates a smaller diameter size.) To reduce mistakes in doses, the syringes used must be calibrated in insulin units/mL—not milliliters (mL) sole-ly, as insulin is prescribed in units. **Use of non-insulin, non-unit-measured syringes cannot be used—they are not interchangeable and can cause under- and/or over-medication administration.** If syringes are multi-use, en-sure they are cleaned, dried, and cared for according to the manufacturer's requirements. And for efficacy and

comfort reasons, never use a dull needle for administration of insulin. **Use of the proper equipment ensures safety, assures that the appropriate amount of insulin is instilled into tissue, and decreases risk of adverse reactions from inappropriately injected insulin.**

7) **For preparation of insulin for administration,** allow insulin to reach room temperature, or follow pharmacy recommendations. Wash hands. After testing blood glucose to determine amount of insulin to inject, fill syringe with that amount of air and inject the air into the vial, after cleansing vial top with alcohol. Then withdraw units to be injected. Ensure no air bubbles are present. To prevent infection, washing hands frequently helps to eliminate contamination. With excess glucose in the body, infection occurs more frequently. Instilling air into the vial eases withdrawal of contents into the syringe. Eliminate air bubbles to help ensure proper amount of insulin will be injected and that the syringe space is not reduced by air and that air will not be injected along with the medication.

8) **Preparation and insulin administration.** Wash hands. Cleanse site with alcohol swab and allow to dry. **Pinch fold of skin, relax muscles, and insert needle at 90° angle into subcutaneous (non-muscle) tissue,** penetrating the skin fold quickly. (If patient is very thin, insert needle at 45° angle.) Do not change direction of needle during insertion or removal: go in and out without turning. Withdraw needle. Messaging of area is detrimental and should not be done, but pressure applied to site is acceptable. **Rotate injection sites often** to prevent hardening of

the skin and other problems, such a dimpling or sunken areas. Use abdomen, upper arms, thighs, and hips as directed by physician. If using the same area of body, ensure at least a one-inch area is maintained between injection sites. Cleansing site and washing hands minimizes risk for infection. Rotating needle once inserted into skin causes discomfort and provides no benefit. Massaging skin changes the route of insulin and causes decreased efficacy. Rotating sites and allowing for injection margins of at least one inch minimizes atrophy of the skin to allow for lifelong injection sites.

9) **Know the signs and symptoms of hypoglycemia which can occur in Type 1 or Type 2 diabetes.** This condition results when there is too little glucose in the blood, typically resulting in an over-administration of insulin or medication, or taking insulin and then not eating, or exercise that was too intense or too long in duration. **Symptoms include headache, vagueness, nervousness, dizziness, uncoordinated movements, paleness (pallor), sweating, palpitations, and fast heart rate (tachycardia). Eventual seizures, loss of consciousness and coma can occur.** If symptoms arise, first test the patient's blood if able. If blood glucose level is low or hypoglycemia is suspected, have patient consume a fast-acting carbohydrate such as orange juice, milk, hard candies, honey, bread/crackers, or other foods containing sugar. Administer to patient's safety and comfort. Call 911 as necessary. In addition, the patient should always have a readily available supply of candy or another sugar source that can be self-administered if the patient suspects possible hypoglycemia.

10) **Meticulous skin care is necessary. Feet should be inspected daily** for small injuries that can be complicated due to decreased blood flow and lack of sensation (neuropathy). Inspect feet while sitting down and hold them up to a mirror to reflect image. This aids in obtaining full view of the soles of the feet, often difficult to visualize. **Never soak feet for any length of time.** Soaking leads to excessive softening of skin (maceration) and promotes infection because the skin is more prone to injury. **Wash and dry skin thoroughly. Blot skin: do not rub.** Drying gently decreases harm to skin yet ensures moisture is removed. **Avoid constricting socks and foot wear.** These decrease blood flow which is already compromised.

11) **Provide full and complete gentle oral care.** Dental hygiene is essential to prevent dryness, gingivitis, and periodontal disease. Obtain professional dental care often, every four to six months, to minimize diabetic complications. Use soft toothbrushes when brushing. Monitor for bad breath, unpleasant tastes, sore, red and/or bleeding gums, and tooth pain, and if these occur, consult your dentist as soon as possible. These could be signs of oral infection and require professional treatment.

12) **Risk for injury increases for the patient** with diabetes due to multiple causes, depending on the progression and stage of the disease. Neuropathies can affect gait and sensation. Visual damage can cause blurred vision, cataracts, and other problems leading to blindness. With variances in glucose in blood, especially hypoglycemia, seizures or altered levels of consciousness can be exhibited. **To prevent injury, ensure rooms are clear of**

**debris. Provide night lights to assist with visualization, especially if vision has been adversely affected.** Patients should always wear protective covering on feet, such as slippers or shoes—socks do not prevent injury. Know the signs and symptoms of hypoglycemia to provide quick treatment and prevent severity. Monitor water temperature to ensure it is not too hot and can cause injury. Neuropathies cause loss of sensation and burns could easily occur without the patent noticing them in time.

13) **Risk for infection increases** in the diabetic patient. Injuries are slower to heal due to decreased blood circulation. In addition, glucose in the blood promotes bacterial growth. Keep nails clean and intact. Monitor for urinary tract infections and yeast infections, especially vaginally and in skin folds. Be protective of feet, even with regard to small cuts or abrasions. **Feet are a likely target for infection due to decreased blood supply,** loss of sensation, and lack of visibility of the soles and outer aspects of feet. **Know the signs and symptoms of infection, which include temperature, pain, malaise, swelling, redness, and discharge.** Consult medical professionals should this occur. Due to underlying diabetes and the effects of the disease, it is not recommended to self-treat infections.

14) **A diabetic diet should be followed by the patient.** This is as individualized to the patient as in his insulin regime. Consultation with medical professionals, a nutritionist, and a dietician is recommended to determine the amount of carbohydrates, proteins, and fats that should be consumed to ensure a balance among caloric intake, energy utilization, and dosing and timing of insulin. **A**

diet that limits sugar, alcohol, salt, and fats is usually recommended. In addition, eating complex carbohydrates decreases sugar levels and, therefore, the amount of insulin that needs to be injected. Caloric intake is often reduced, especially in the obese patient. Foods that promote satiation (feeling of fullness), especially those high in fiber, are suggested. A food-exchange program is often taught which allows the patient to select set amounts of food, based upon specific patient parameters, from basic food groups to allow for independence, as well as teaching skills in reading food labels. **Dietary changes can greatly increase the efficacy of medications as well as leading to better quality of life in general.** Professionals can pinpoint specifics and knowledge in label reading can bring hidden bad ingredients to the forefront. Consultation with professionals can provide eating strategies and options that may be overlooked by a layman. This then increases compliance and makes eating a pleasure rather than a diet.

15) **Maintain records of tested blood glucose levels, insulin injected (including time administered, type, and amount given), and diet/foods eaten.** Records provide means for medical professionals to evaluate treatment regime. They also enhance the participation and compliance of the patience by having "to do" and "record" actions.

16) **Patient concerns include a lack of independence, an altered self-image, fear of economic loss due to illness or loss of work, coping with a chronic illness, and/or fear of complications.** With diabetes, more frequent visits to

medical professionals will be required. One is no longer free to do what and when he desires and may feel trapped by medication administration and dietary constraints. With additional medications and doctor visits, funds may be depleted. Fear of complications and living with a chronic illness can seem daunting for a newly diagnosed diabetic patient, especially when outward signs and symptoms of the disease may not have presented yet. All of these are genuine concerns and realistic losses to the patient. **However, with patience and teaching, the patient becomes more aware and self-motivated.** Control over the disease increases. Over time, he will probably feel better, which also leads to continued compliance. Stress the benefits, his accomplishments. Allow for frustration and disappointment. Backward steps may occur, but with encouragement, they will hopefully be few and progress will continue.

# CHAPTER 16

# REPRODUCTIVE AND URINARY SYSTEMS

**The organs and functioning units in the reproductive system differ between males and females.** While the basic function of the system, whether male or female, is to produce reproductive cells, gametes; males produce them by way of testes and females via ovaries.

**Regardless of the sex, both reproductive systems require tubes by which the gametes are transported for the union of sperm and eggs (ova) for fertilization** and formation of a new organism.

The male reproductive system includes the penis, vas deferens, testes which produce sperm, and glands which secrete fluids and hormones for the reproductive task.

The female reproductive system includes the vagina and vaginal canal, fallopian tubes, ovaries which produce ova, uterus, and glands which secrete different hormones and fluids, in a similar fashion necessary for reproduction.

**The reproductive system is often assessed with the urinary system. In fact, portions of the reproductive system are**

combined with the urinary system. This is termed the uro-genital system.

**Numerous disorders can occur in the reproductive system.** They are often related to cancer, such as ovarian, uterine, testicular, for example. Other problems result in infection or excessive growth of glands such as the prostate, as exhibited with prostatitis and benign prostatic hyperplasia (BPH), respectively, in males, causing difficulties in urination, for example. Females often exhibit problems and disorders with menstruation when abnormal and excessive uterine bleeding, lack of menstruation, (amenorrhea) or painful menstruation (dysmenorrhea).

Many disorders and problems affecting the reproductive system require surgical intervention. Once the dysfunctional organ is excised (removed), home care considerations then relate to post-surgical care, which includes assessing for signs and symptoms of infection, promoting healing, and allowing time to return to normal function.

## Reproduction

Reproduction is the process by which new life is formed. While the method is very different for plants versus animals, the outcome is the same. The purpose of reproduction is to produce new life to ensure the species not only continues, but thrives. Genetic material is passed down from generation to generation. However, duplication is not the sole purpose. Replication of the species' best properties are passed down and changes to the genetic material are made over time to propagate and enhance the entities, resulting in increased chances of survival as well as a stronger, and sometimes more advanced organism.

In humans, the goal of reproduction is to produce children who are biological descendants, as well as cultural, traditional, and familial offspring. This is accomplished by a union of male and female genetic material brought together via sexual reproduction. To complete this task, although the two sexes have different anatomy and function independently, they work together (synergistically) to obtain one outcome: fertilization of reproductive cells (gametes) for formation of a new organism.

**Gametes include sperm in males and eggs (ova) in females.** Both sexes have structures (gonads) that produce gametes, with tubes and ducts for gamete transportation, and glands which secrete substances to support and enhance survival of the gametes and fertilization.

**In males,** the gonads that continually produce sperm throughout a male's lifetime are the testes. Testes are dual oval-shaped glands which also have cells producing fluids to nourish sperm and others which produce the hormone testosterone. The testes are held in place by the scrotum which functions to adjust the temperature within the testes necessary for sperm viability and development. Muscles in this tissue contract with decreased temperature to bring these organs closer to the body to provide warmth. In contrast, these muscles also relax to lower them from the pelvis for cooling.

**Mature sperm are transported** to and stored by the ductus deferens (also called the vas deferens) which also functions to force sperm to a portion of the urethra (the prostatic urethra) during ejaculation via the penis. Other accessory sex glands produce and secrete substances that form semen, the liquid portion of ejaculated fluid that does not include sperm. Semen provides a substance for sperm transportation and motility as well as neutralizing fluids to promote their viability to increase chances of fertilization.

**In females**, the gonads that produce eggs ("ova": singular is "ovum") are the ovaries. Similar to male testes, these are dual almond-shaped glands but contained within the body; they store and mature ova prior to their release during ovulation. Historically it was believed that ova are not constantly produced and that the number present at birth remains static until death. This is the opposite of sperm production. However, some evidence suggests that this may not be the case but has yet to be determined conclusively.

**The ovaries also secrete the hormones estrogen and progesterone** to assist in the maturation process of an ovum along with other hormones, as well as prepare the female body for implantation if fertilization should occur. Once an ovum has matured and is released from an ovary, it is transported via the uterine (or fallopian) tubes, where fertilization by sperm usually occurs, to the uterus. Regardless of whether the ovum was fertilized, the fallopian tubes provides the route for the egg to reach the uterus.

**If the ovum is fertilized,** it will implant itself in the uterine wall for growth, maturation, and development into an embryo and later, a fetus. If unfertilized, it will eventually be discarded with uterine tissues during **menstruation**. The vagina is basically a structural passage that allows transport into and out of the uterus. Sperm moves from the penis into the vagina during intercourse. Sperm then proceeds into the uterus into the fallopian tubes to fertilize ova. If the ovum is fertilized, during birth it serves as part of the birth canal. If fertilization does not take place, the vagina functions to eliminate and evacuate uterine blood and tissues during menstruation.

In addition to the overview of the structure and function of the male and female reproductive system presented here, **there are other structures which have not been described.** In addition, disease process and illnesses are also not addressed, as many interventions are dictated around medications or surgical procedures. Lastly, although this system is often addressed and assessed in conjunction with the urinary system; nevertheless, they are two very distinct and separate systems.

**In this section, urinary disorders will be addressed.**

While the digestive system's large colon eliminates solid waste, **the urinary system functions in a similar capacity in the removal of liquid waste via the kidneys.** By using a complex method of filtration, various tubes throughout the system capture and retain needed bodily fluid, minerals, and electrolytes, and the remaining fluid and non-essential substances are stored in the bladder to be later excreted as urine. **In addition, the system helps to regulate calcium and the acid-base (pH) balance of the body.**

**The urinary system is comprised** of the kidneys (to regulate the amount and composition of the blood by producing urine), ureters (to move urine from the kidneys), bladder (to hold and store urine received from the ureters), and urethra (to release urine from the bladder for elimination outside the body). While the functional elements of the urinary system do not differ between males and females, the length of the urethra does. Therefore, **females are more prone to urinary tract infections.**

**The kidneys are the main organ of this system** and are comprised of small units (nephrons) that filter the body's blood. Besides maintaining fluid balance by eliminating excess water, they perform many other functions. They regulate the composition of fluid by removing or retaining various electrolytes such as hydrogen, sodium, potassium, chlorine, and regulate the body's pH within a small range of 7.37 to 7.43. Too much retained hydrogen results in metabolic acidosis; too little results in metabolic alkalosis.

**By regulating the amount of water that is retained in the body, the kidneys assist in the regulation of blood pressure. This system also produces erythropoietin when the body's blood oxygen supply is decreased. This hormone then prompts the bone marrow to produce red blood cells. Also, they synthesize vitamin D.**

**Disorders of the renal (kidney) system can be acute or chronic.** The severity dictates whether measures are required to provide or enhance elimination of urine, as well as provide filtering of the blood. **Acute renal failure** can resolve and normal function may resume. **Chronic renal failure** is irreversible and may require **dialysis** to remove toxins and fluid that the kidneys are no longer able to remove via filtration.

**Hyperplasia (abnormal growth) of the prostate gland in males** can restrict urine to pass, causing a feeling of urgency, a slow stream, and incomplete evacuation of the bladder. Medication often enhances flow but at times surgical intervention is necessary. Other methods of urinary elimination may take the form of catheters or surgical urinary diversions.

Some of the various urinary system conditions and care considerations that may be experienced in the home-care setting appear below.

**Chronic Renal (Kidney) Disease:** is caused by a gradual and prolonged destruction of nephrons, which results in the inability to filter sufficient fluid and waste from the blood. This disease often results from infection, diabetes, or high blood pressure. As the amount of functioning nephrons declines, filtering the blood of toxins and waste decreases as well. At the point at which most nephrons no longer function and the substances in the blood that are normally filtered and excreted by the kidneys remain, **uremia** results, a toxic situation causing harmful conditions in many other bodily systems. At this point, because the kidneys no longer are functioning sufficiently, **dialysis is usually necessary** to remove excess fluid and toxins from the blood.

**Excess fluid in the blood (hypervolemia)** can contribute to cardiac problems such as increases in blood pressure and pulses, or lead to congestive heart failure. Respiratory complications are evidenced by crackles (a type of adventitious lung sounds) or life-threatening pulmonary edema. Generalized edema is noted in feet, ankles and puffiness around the eyes. However, the opposite is also possible, and too much water is lost by lack of reabsorption **(hypovolemia)**. This can lead to dry and scaling skin, hair, and nails, and lack of skin turgor (firmness).

**Waste build-up in the blood causes retention of potassium (hyperkalemia) which can cause cardiac arrhythmias, malaise, muscle cramping, paralysis, and even cardiac arrest.** Increases in phosphate (hyperphosphatemia) caused by decreased excretion can also lead to cardiovascular risks.

**Anemia** results from lack of red blood cell production when erythropoietin is no longer synthesized. **Weak bones** (osteomalacia) occurs due to lack of calcium (hypocalcemia) caused by a decrease in the synthesis of vitamin D by the kidneys.

**Azotemia** results when there is an accumulation of nitrogen and urea which are the products of protein metabolism. As wastes build up, the GI system is also affected, presenting as nausea, vomiting, anorexia, and abdominal pain. Neurological symptoms appear as confusion, altered levels of consciousness and mentation.

**Acute Renal Failure:** is the sudden loss of kidney function. It may result from the obstruction of blood or from trauma resulting in decreased blood flow to the kidneys, damage to the filtering structures within the kidneys due to toxins or infection, or obstruction of urine outflow. Often this condition is reversible with the return of most, if not all, kidney function. Primary treatment is the reversal of the failure's cause.

**Regardless of the cause, the acute disease progression can result in the same or similar symptoms as the chronic disease.** The severity, length, and course of the illness will depend on the damage incurred as well as on the underlying cause. **Typically, however, the healing and recovery process will follow three paths or phases.** The first phase is the oliguric phase, and during this time there is a decrease in urine secretion. The diuretic phase is the opposite. During this second phase, urine output is greatly increased. The last phase is the recovery phase. It is in this phase that normal function gradually returns, with the elimination of wastes and fluid. **However, if the underlying cause of the acute condition is not reversed, chronic renal disease could follow.**

*Care Considerations for Chronic Renal Disease and Acute Renal Failure:*

1) **Primarily dietary changes are required for both diseases.** However, the acute illness should be temporary and care involves supportive actions. Conversely, the chronic disease usually increases in severity with the potential of requiring artificial blood filtering (dialysis).

2) Depending on the stage of the disease, patients should consume **low-protein diets** to decrease protein metabolism and the byproducts that the kidneys can't excrete.

3) **Electrolyte balance is necessary** because the kidneys are no longer able to remove these from the blood, and excesses of some can be damaging to the body, even deadly. **In particular, the amounts of potassium and phosphorus require monitoring,** and foods that are plentiful in these substances should be avoided. Some medications are available to bind electrolytes to decrease their availability in the blood and make elimination easier.

4) **Fluid intake should be restricted** as in later of stages of the disease, oliguria (decreased urination) or anuria (inability to urinate) result. Restricting fluid prevents fluid overload, and this can decrease risks for high blood pressure, edema, and pulmonary overload.

5) **Monitor and record fluid intake and output.** Recording both provides indication of fluid retention in the body. Daily weights can also provide insight with respect to excess fluid in the body.

6) **Restrict sodium** to decrease water retention.

7) **Assess for signs and symptoms of uremia** caused by nitrogen substances that are retained in the body. Symptoms include dizziness, nausea, vomiting, coma, convulsions, hypertension, hard rapid pulse, dry skin, oliguria or anuria, odor of urine on the breath or in perspirations. Treatment often requires **dialysis**.

8) Due to **weakness** from toxin build-up or increased fluid retention, mobility could be an issue. Perform **range of motion** exercise and position changes. **Safety measures** include neurological assessments for dizziness or confusion (altered mentation) as well as muscle fatigue, cramping, and weakness from excess potassium.

9) **Administer medications as ordered**. Numerous drugs assist in the conditions associated with kidney disease. **Anti-hypertensives** are prescribed to lower blood pressure. **Diuretics** are taken to promote urination and decrease fluid retention when the ability to void is present. **Anti-emetics** are used to decrease nausea, vomiting, and gastrointestinal irritation. **Laxatives and stool softeners** are used to promote bowel elimination which can be a secondary problem due to lack of fluids, limited mobility, and dietary changes. **Iron supplements** may be used to combat anemia. **Synthetic erythropoietin** may be injected to promote formation of red blood cells. If this is ineffectual, **blood transfusions** may be required. **Anti-pruritics** are administered to relieve itching (pruritus) that often results from dry skin. **Electrolyte binding medications** may be given to decrease serum phosphate

or potassium levels. These medications will not provide a cure to the disease, but can relieve adverse symptoms associated with it.

10) **During the end stage of the disease**, some form of **dialysis** is most often required.

**Dialysis:** is required during the most severe and final stage of kidney disease (end-stage renal disease). Dialysis is performed to remove fluid and toxins that the kidneys would normal filter, resorb, and excrete from the body. The two most common types of dialysis are **hemodialysis and peritoneal dialysis**. Whichever method is used, this treatment will continue throughout the life of the patient or until a kidney transplant is performed.

**Hemodialysis** (HD) filters the blood and is accomplished by a machine that removes "dirty" blood from the body, filters it via a semi-permeable membrane to eliminate toxic materials and electrolytes as well as to maintain proper fluid levels and acid-base balances. "Clean" blood is then returned to the body. This type of dialysis requires a surgically made connection or passage (fistula) between a vein and an artery, usually created in the upper extremity, called an arteriovenous (AV) fistula. Often dialysis is performed at an outside, dedicated dialysis facility three times a week, with each session lasting roughly 4 hours.

**Peritoneal dialysis** (PD), although providing the same outcome, uses the peritoneal cavity as the filtering membrane. A permanent catheter is implanted into the abdomen to instill a warm, sterile dialyzing chemical solution into the peritoneal cavity. The solution remains for a prescribed amount of time and is then removed. This process could take place overnight or throughout the day at regular intervals. The advantages to this type of dialysis are the ability to perform the action individually, and not having to rely on outside intervention or long-lasting appointments. However, infection at the catheter site or peritonitis can be complications.

### *Care Considerations for Hemodialysis and Peritoneal Dialysis:*

1) **Hemodialysis (HD)** uses a surgially fashioned AV (arteriovenous) fistula or AV graft. This is created under the skin with no outside route that can lead to infection. However, during the dialysis process, needles are inserted and strict aseptic technique is required to prevent infection.

2) The **HD fistula** and the extremity in which it is placed require caution, care, and watchfulness to protect that extremity and fistula. That fistula or graft provides life to the patient. Blood pressure readings, tight clothing, injury, and blood sampling should not be performed on that arm.

3) **Peritoneal dialysis (PD)** requires strict aseptic technique to perform the procedure. In addition, dexterity and eyesight is necessary to perform the connections of the dialysis solution to the catheter while maintaining sterility.

4) **The patient using PD** needs to adjust his lifestyle to coincide with the dialysis process. This includes adjusting medication scheduling to coincide with the PD process, especially if it is performed at different intervals on different days, as well as allowing sufficient time for the

instilled solution to remain to complete filtration. After the solution is instilled, a bloating, full, uncomfortable feeling can be exhibited. However, the solution must not be prematurely drained. If the solution is instilled at night time during sleep, changes to the bedroom and sleeping routines may be required.

5) Proper care to the **PD catheter** is required. The site should be assessed for inflammation and infection daily. If infection is suspected, obtain medical assistance.

6) Assess for signs and symptoms of **peritonitis with PD.** This can potentially be a life-threatening condition. Symptoms include chill, fever, fast heart rate (tachycardia), abdominal pain or distention, respiratory difficulty due to decreased effort related to the pain, vomiting, and low blood pressure (hypotension). Seek medical assistance immediately.

**Urinary Diversions:** are surgical procedures creating reservoirs for holding urine. In these procedures, the kidneys function within normal limits. However, the elimination of urine does not occur due to trauma or cancer of the bladder or urethra, for example. Urine is merely rerouted and bypasses the bladder and urethra. **There are two types of urinary diversions: continent diversions and incontinent diversions.** Both types require the patient to be sufficiently dexterous to either perform a sterile catheterization or change outside appliances.

**Continent diversions** are internal pouches created from a portion of the large intestine. A stoma is created with a closure piece that is similar to a valve that can be opened or closed at will. This eliminates urine leakage. The reservoir is internal but self-catheterization is required to empty urine from the pouch, and this is required approximately four to six times per day. In addition, because the pouch is created from a segment of the large intestine, which produces mucus to aid in stool elimination, the reservoir requires irrigation to decrease potential for blockage from the mucus. However, there are no outside bags to collect urine, no leakage, and clothes can be protected with the use of a small piece of gauze to trap mucus. Sterile technique is required during the procedure.

**Incontinent diversions** are similar to colostomies which reroute stool from the colon to an outside collection appliance. The difference is that urine is collected. With this type of diversion, there is an opening directly to the abdominal wall. Appliances are required at all times and the bags must be emptied frequently. However, there is no sterile technique required and no irrigation. The bag is held in place, again similar to colostomies, by adhesives. But these can be irritating to the body.

*Care Considerations for Continent Urinary Diversions:*

1) **Sterile technique is required when emptying the pouch during catheterization**. It is also essential to clean the site before and after the procedure. Before catheterizing (or intubation), clean the stoma in outward circular motions with a prescribed cleansing agent (such as providone-iodine). When done emptying the pouch, again clean with gauze and liquid soap, rinse, and pat dry. Care to the stoma and nearby (peristomal) skin as well as sterile technique is essential to maintenance of the device and to minimize risk of infection.

2) **Before inserting catheter**, lubricate with a water-soluble lubricant. Using petroleum-based products increases risk of infection. Lubrication also decreases damage to the valve when inserting the catheter. Gently insert the catheter using a rolling motion in minimize damage, and continue until urine flows. Taking deep breaths during insertion or changing positions can aid in inserting the catheter if resistance is felt.

3) **During irrigation**, after emptying the pouch at regular intervals, irrigate and instill sterile normal saline. The amount and time frames when this is required should be prescribed. Irrigation is required to prevent blockage that can occur due to the mucus produced by the large intestines. The saline will drain with gravity.

4) **Before the catheter is removed** from the valve, patient should cough a few times. This will help expel residual urine and/or normal saline from the pouch.

5) **After intubation catheter use**, clean as recommended by manufacturer or physician, or discard if single-use only. If reusable, be sure to rinse well to clear all mucus.

6) **Ensure a catheter is always available** and ready to use. Keep track of intubations to ensure the reservoir does not become too full. In time the size of the pouch will increase. Damage to the reservoir or urine leakage could occur with too much urine volume.

7) **Body image disturbances** are common, especially after initial creation. Provide encouragement, supportive

communication, and patience. Offer assistance with tracking intubation times and provide gentle reminders if necessary. Allow patient to express difficulties and vent frustrations but direct him to positive outcomes.

### Care Considerations for Incontinent Urinary Diversions:

1) **When applying new ring and appliance,** ensure that measurements of the stoma compared to the outside appliance ring and pouch are within a small margin for proper placement around the stoma. This is usually 1/16 to 1/8 of an inch. If the ring is too large, leakage may happen. If it is too small, damage to the stoma could occur.

2) **After emptying the pouch**, cleanse the stoma and area with soap and water. Pat the skin dry to decrease possible irritation. Apply skin preparations, if so advised, to help adhere appliance and provide protective barrier to the skin. Then apply ring and appliance and hold in place to ensure a solid seal.

3) **At night**, the pouch can be connected to a drainage bag for continuous removal via gravity. This helps to eliminate leakage or build-up of urine that can create difficulties during sleep when volume is not attended to.

4) **Body image disturbances** are common especially after initial creation. Provide encouragement, supportive communication, and patience. Offer to assist with measuring appliance and skin care. Allow patient to express difficulties and vent frustrations but direct him to positive outcomes.

**Urinary Catheterization:** is performed to allow urine to flow from the bladder for elimination outside the body. This may be required when spinal cord injuries prevent normal voiding due to loss of function from spinal nerve damage. Often fully incontinent patients are catheterized to prevent spontaneous voiding which could cause damage to skin due to moisture and the acidic nature of urine. Other times, it is done to provide a "normal" lifestyle. Besides providing a means to eliminate and collect urine, sterile urine sampling can be obtained for diagnostic testing related to urinary tract infections, for example. **There are many types of catheters that can be used.** These include indwelling bladder catheters, intermittent catheterization, and condom catheters for males.

**Indwelling catheters** are often used in hospital and nursing home settings due to incontinence, but are also used when obstruction prevents normal urination. These catheters are inserted into the urethra up to the bladder. After placement is established by the flow of urine, sterile normal saline is inserted into a balloon to hold the device in place. Urine is then eliminated via gravity into a collection bag. **Risk for infection can be high** during placement as well as during the time the catheter is in place. In some cases, kidney disease can result due to upward moving infections that traveled along the catheter to the bladder eventually affecting the kidneys.

**Intermittent catheters** are preferred to indwelling catheters, which cause increased risk of infection to the urinary tract. However, catheterization is required often, and this increases the infection risk during each insertion. This form of catheterization is often necessary for paraplegics and individuals with spinal cord injuries. Although there is no obstruction of the urethra, signals from the brain are blocked and prevent normal voiding.

A **condom catheter** is specific to incontinent males. As the name suggests, a condom-like apparatus is place over the penis and urine flows from the condom via tubing to a collection bag that is placed on the leg. There is virtually no loss of mobility. Although risk for infection always exists, there is no invasive procedure to the sterile bladder cavity. The bag is emptied when approximately half full. There is, unfortunately, no similar solution for females.

### Care Considerations for Urinary Catheterization:

1) **All catheters are vulnerable to urinary tract infections** that may result during placement or dwell time. Strict sterile technique is required for placement, without exception, as the urinary system is a sterile one and is easily contaminated. Infections in the bladder, for example, can progress upward to the kidneys and cause irreparable harm to kidney function. In addition, extreme results can result in septicemia which is an infection that spreads to the blood.

2) Whether an intermittent or indwelling catheter is placed, consideration is required concerning the sex of the patient. **The male patient's urethra is very long and typically extends approximately 12 to 13 inches before reaching the bladder. In contrast, the female urethra is only about 5 inches in length.** Continue to slowly progress the catheter until urine is expelled, using sterile technique during the entire time. Stopping and restarting the

procedure prolongs discomfort and increases the risk for infection.

3) The patient will normally experience pressure and discomfort during the process if sensations are recognized. In addition, often the bladder is distended which causes discomfort itself. Deep breaths will help advance the catheter. **Ensure sufficient lubrication is provided on the catheter before insertion.** Relief will be felt immediately upon entering the bladder.

4) **If the patient is an uncircumcised male**, the penis foreskin must be pulled back. Ensure that the foreskin is replaced and returned to the original position prior to the catheterization. Retracted foreskin can cause damage due to potential lack of blood supply to the organ.

5) **Once the catheter enters the bladder, urine will flow.** Normal voiding occurs when the bladder contains approximately 250mL. The maximum immediate outflow of urine after catheterization should be no more than 1000mL. Exceeding this amount can cause detrimental fluid shifts within the body.

6) If an **indwelling catheter** is placed, remove it as soon as possible to decrease risk for infection.

# CHAPTER 17

# INTEGUMENTARY (SKIN) SYSTEM

Often the forgotten child, **the skin system makes up more of the body than any other system.** From its uppermost tissue layer (epidermis) to the various layers beneath it, the skin is involved in many functions.

**Besides the skin, this system also includes oil (sebaceous) and sweat (sudoriferous) glands, and nerve receptors.** It also gives rise to hair and nails. **However, the primary function of skin is defense.** It provides the boundary to prohibit or discourage foreign substances from entering the body. When compromised with a cut or scrape, it utilizes defenses to repair the impaired barrier to protect and promote healing.

**While covering and protecting the body in multiple layers, the integumentary system regulates temperature (thermoregulation) during perspiration or shivering.** Temperature regulation and excretion are performed by means of sweat. The skin also plays an integral role in the **vitamin D synthesis** necessary for calcium absorption essential for skeletal formation and mainte-nance, and cardiac function.

Derived from the Latin word "integumentum" meaning "covering", the integumentary system is comprised of the skin and all its associated elements, such as nails, hair, and glands. While the skin furnishes an outer form to house the internal works of the body, it provides so much more.

The chief organ in this system is the skin. Organs are often perceived as being internal structures. They may be individual and located in one part of the body, such as the heart or brain. Other times, organs appear in pairs but are found in close proximity to each other, such as the kidneys and lungs. Organs may be small and held in the palm of a hand, such as an eye which is about one inch in size, or large, as exampled by the small intestine which may exceed 19 feet.

The skin's primary function is as a physical barrier between the environment and the body. It is the rock walls that guard the perimeter of the kingdom. When unharmed and unbroken by cuts or abrasions, it prevents most infectious agents (pathogens), such as bacteria, from entering the body. This is accomplished by the many layers of tissues that compose it. However, when harmed by infection for example, the skin initiates repair by means of an inflammatory process.

The outermost or top layer (epidermis) of the skin is four or five layers in thickness. It is constantly renewed and replaced, and essentially "dead" at the outermost surface. The cell turnover in a year can be eight pounds. Yet, it provides immunity, heat, prevention or promotion of water loss, and UV light protection. It also contains various cell types at lower levels to provide water-proofing and touch sensation. In addition, there are pores for hair follicles and sweat (sudoriferous) glands. Structures, such as fingernails, are also created by the epidermis.

**The inner layer (dermis) usually has two layers which contain collagen and elastin fibers for strength, hair follicles with attached oil (sebaceous) glands, nerve roots and endings, and blood vessels.** Variances in thickness occur depending on the location; they may be very thin, such as on the eyelids, or thick, such as on the soles of the feet.

**There are two types of skin,** which differ in their thickness, amount of blood vessels, nerve supply, gland types, skin strength, and absence of hair. The majority of the body is made of skin that is considered thin and contains hair, such as the face, arms, legs, trunk, and pubic area. While the amount or coarseness of this hair may vary, they all contain hair. **Hair is protective: the scalp protects from sun and injury; eyebrows and eyelashes protect from foreign particles, and nostril hair protects from inhaling foreign particles and insects, for example.** Along with hair are oil (sebaceous) glands connected to hair follicles. **Sebaceous glands** protect the hair from drying by preventing excess water evaporation from the skin surface, and protect from bacterial growth while keeping skin soft and resilient. Skin that is thick and hairless appears on the palms of the hand and soles of the feet, for example, where friction and wear are greatest.

**In addition to protection, however, another major function of the skin is temperature regulation (thermoregulation).** This is accomplished by blood vessels and sweat (sudoriferous) glands which have receptors in the dermis to regulate secretion. During high temperatures, water and internal heat are released via sweat glands. The evaporation of fluid (sweat, perspiration) cools the body. When temperatures are low, sweat production is decreased and heat is conserved. The skin's blood supply, which is quite extensive, works in a similar manner. The small arterial vessels (arterioles) expand to help dissipate heat and during levels of moderate exercise. However, the vessels will also constrict during cold periods to protect the internal organs, as well as direct blood flow into muscles during strenuous exercise.

**Sudoriferous glands empty onto the skin surface via pores,** and besides providing sweat for evaporation and cooling, small amounts of wastes are excreted. Waste material includes salt, urea, glucose, lactic acid, and other organic compounds.

**Lastly, the skin serves to provide tactile stimulation as well as absorption, synthesis and storage of vitamin D.** The sense of touch is accomplished by the skin via nerve endings and receptors. These detect stimuli such as pain, pressure, touch, and heat, causing automatic reflexes to pull away or change an action, if it is a negative stimulus. Touch, providing an ability to grasp, hold, and discern textures, especially in the hands, along with fine motor skills, allows for dexterity and use for numerous circumstances and actions. From sun exposure (UVB rays) the skin produces vitamin D, and the derivatives needed by the body are synthesized by the liver and kidneys. Ultimately, this substance is changed to a product that aids in calcium absorption, essential for the skeletal system and various calcium-sensitive mechanisms that regulate internal functions via ion exchanges, such as heart beats.

While the skin is a very large and multi-functioning organ of the body, nursing services do not usually dictate long-term requirements. The exception to this is **pressure ulcers.** Although discussed in other sections of this book, they will also be addressed here.

**Pressure Injuries:** previously called "pressure" or "decubitus" ulcers, commonly referred to as **"bedsores,"** these are defined as **areas where skin death occurs because it is compressed between an internal bony projection and another external surface, such as a chair or bed, for a period of time.** The injury results from the pressure exerted on the skin which lies between the two objects. As the internal bone pushes against a hard, external surface, the skin covering the bone becomes damaged. This is due to loss of oxygen because a constant flow of blood is restricted. Besides a deficiency of blood flow to the tissues, the patient's underlying health condition, such as nutrition and sensory perception, as well as additional factors such as moisture, friction, and shear are also contributing factors causing skin damage.

**The bony projections, or prominences, that most often initiate this damage include the sacrum (which lies at the base of the spinal column), the heel of the foot, elbow, outer ankle bone (lateral malleolus), outer hip bone (greater trochanter), and projections of the hip bone (ischial tuberosity).** The patient's position could be that of sitting in a chair or lying in bed. **Skin damage could result in two or three hours or as little as 90 minutes depending on the force of pressure force in addition to the patient's pressure tolerance and tissue health.**

**Staging is used to characterize the extent of the injury and to dictate protocols for healing.** Staging is evaluated visually by using the National Pressure Ulcer Advisory Panel (NPUAP) per their 2016 guidelines. If eschar (dead, dried, brown-blackish crust) or slough (dead, mucus-like, yellow, gray, green material) is present, the wound cannot be accurately staged until the substance is removed. In addition, location of the wound is pivotal. Some areas of the body, such as the bridge of the nose or the ankles, do not have a lot of subcutaneous tissue. In such locations, the wound beds themselves may be shallow in comparison with other areas of the body.

*Stage 1 Pressure Injury* is "non-blanchable erythema of intact skin." It indicates an area of redness (erythema) in light-pigmented skin or an area that is darker in dark-pigmented skin. When a finger is pressed against this tissue and quickly released, the fingerprint area returns immediately to the original skin color; if it does not, it is non-blanchable. Edema and tissue hardness may also present. But the skin is intact and there is no outward injury except for redness.

*Stage 2 Pressure Injury* is "partial-thickness skin loss with exposed dermis." Tissue damage to the layers of the epidermis and/or dermis is evident. It is superficial and may look like an abrasion, blister, or shallow crater. Actual injury to the skin is apparent.

*Stage 3 Pressure Injury* is much more severe and termed "full thickness with skin loss". There is full skin damage and loss extends to tissues that lie under the skin (subcutaneous tissue) including fat (adipose) tissue. Evident injury is without question. At times the edges of the wound roll back (epibole) creating undermining of the pressure wound that is hidden by the upper rolled-back skin, making the wound appear smaller than it actually is. The wound bed may have tunneling, when open passages extend further into the tissue. Often deep craters are formed.

**Stage 4 Pressure Injury**, "full-thickness skin and tissue loss" is the most severe stage of pressure wound. Tissue loss and death are extensive continuing into the deep tissues. Muscle, bone, and supporting structures such as tendons are often visible. Epibole (undermining) and tunneling are often present. Osteomyelitis, a severe skeletal infection, may occur.

**A patient's risk for pressure wounds can be assessed using various scales. One often used is the Braden Scale.** It measures six specific areas that may predict the potential occurrence of a pressure wound. Categories include:

1) **Sensory perception**—is the patient able to recognize pressure on a part of his body?

2) **Moisture**—is his skin often wet or usually dry?

3) **Activity**—is the patient bedridden or physically active?

4) **Mobility**—is the patient paralyzed and requires assistance for body changes or can he change his body's position at will?

5) **Nutrition**—is the patient receiving sufficient nutrition; are most meals eaten or often does he not eat?

6) **Friction and shear**—in caring for and positioning the patient, is sliding on the sheets an occurrence, does the patient frequently slide down in the bed due to gravity

and often needs positioning, or does he have the muscle strength to lift his body to position himself and usually maintains a position that does not result in sliding down?

**Each category is given a value of one to four (except category six which has a total of three). The lower the number, the more prone the patient may suffer injury.** For example, a score of "one" in the categories of "moisture" and "mobility" would be assigned to a patient that is "constantly moist" and "bedfast." Conversely, a score of "four" would be given if the patient is "rarely moist" and "walks frequently." **Scores for all six areas are totaled. The highest possible score is 23.** If the patient's score is 17 to 23, the patient is at little to no risk. A score less than or equal to 16 indicates there is certain risk for the patient. A patient at high risk has a total score less than or equal to nine.

**Using this scale is simply an indication of risk.** If the patient has a high score, pressure wounds could still occur. However, they are just less likely to happen. These are merely tools to help assess the patient's needs and requirements to prevent formation of pressure ulcers.

*Care Considerations for Pressure Injuries:*

1) **The best care is that in which a pressure injury does not develop.** Unfortunately, sometimes even though superlative care is provided, a pressure injury will result. However, there are steps that can be taken to minimize possible occurrence of these wounds.

2) **When bathing, use mild soap and warm water.** Harsh

perfumed soaps and hot water can be drying, irritate skin, or actually cause damage.

3) **Use a moisturizer after cleansing.** These help seal skin to prevent moisture loss. Avoid products that are thick and do not absorb well, as these tend to prohibit the skin's natural ability to breathe.

4) **Keep the patient dry.** If the patient is incontinent, perform frequent (disposable) undergarment changes every 3 or 4 hours, or more often if needed. Use a skin-protecting barrier, such as A+D ointment to provide a shield between caustic urine and stool, as well as protecting from moisture in general. Specialized water-proof pads are available to provide an additional barrier. Use those made from cloth, not plastic, so the skin's ability to breathe is maintained.

5) **Turn and position the patient every two hours.** Use variations of all four possible positions as can be tolerated: side-lying (lateral, left and right), on back (supine), and on stomach (prone). The more positions used, the more time a patient has to enhance blood flow to rested areas. Rather than have the patient be at a right angle to the mattress when on his side, utilizing a 30-degree lateral position using pillows for support and protection minimizes direct contact with bony prominences.

6) **Keep head of bed at a thirty-degree angle as much as possible.** If the head is higher, shearing forces caused by sliding greatly increase.

7) **Range of motion exercises aid in blood flow as well as prevent contractures.**

8) **Ensure sufficient nutrition and fluids.** Offer a variety of easy-to-digest, healthy foods, including protein to sustain muscle mass and promote healthy skin. Provide more frequent and smaller meals throughout the day; this can be less intimidating to the patient. More may be consumed in many small meals than in three larger ones. If the patient is unwilling or unable to eat a sufficient amount, numerous liquid supplements are available on the market to bridge the protein/nutrition gap. In addition, for patients that are unable to eat orally and utilize a gastric tube for nutrition, consult a medical professional. Many formulas are available via prescription, and a medical professional will be able to suggest one that is best for the patient's needs.

9) **Check skin often, especially in areas of bony prominences.** If injury is suspected but the skin remains blanchable, other skin assessments and evidence may suggest breakdown. Compare that area to the skin that surrounds it. **Some danger signs:** The skin itself may be taut or shiny. The temperature may be warmer initially, but later stages may present as cooler. The texture may be different and appear rippled like an orange peel. The area may feel more spongy or, perhaps, firm and hard. Looking for subtle changes in the skin can promote immediate corrective action to halt the progression of the wound and limit further injury.

10) **If injury should appear, it is best to consult with a**

**medical professional, such as a specialized Wound Care Nurse, to treat the wound.** Depending on the stage of the wound, various protocols and equipment will be utilized. Specific determinations need to be made concerning the best method for healing. For example, a clean wound base is essential for healing. Cleaning solutions generally include normal saline but other commercial products are also available. One that is effective but not damaging to the tissue is required. Medications may be applied to the wound, such as ointments that debride dead tissue or slough. Besides ointments and creams, wound beds may sometimes require mechanical or chemical debridement. Dressing will be applied to the pressure injuries. There are many types of dressings as well as many methods of application and use. For example, a dry dressing is used when drainage is minimal, to inhibit bacteria, and to prevent further injury. Moist dressings aid in full-thickness, crater-like wounds. Wet-to-dry dressings are used for debridement. A wet dressing is placed directly on the wound bed. It draws out and picks up pus (exudate) and other debris present in the wound. As the dressing dries, the wound material adheres to the dressing. When the dressing is removed, it pulls the wound contents out with it. A dry dressing is placed over the wet one to merely protect from bacteria. In addition, as the injury begins healing, so will the course of treatment. Lastly, most usually, all wound beds are colonized with bacteria. Swabbing the wound bed will provide a diagnosis of the organisms to ensure the efficacy of prescribed antibiotics, if necessary, will be appropriate. As the complexity of this section illustrates, wound care requires involvement of a medical professional.

# CHAPTER 18

# MUSCULOSKELETAL SYSTEM

The skeletal system is inter-related with the muscular system and both are often assessed simultaneously.

**The skeletal system is the framework of the body. It is comprised of the bones, of which there are 80 in the trunk and 126 in the limbs for a total of 206 bones in the body, as well as joints, and ligaments which attach the joints to the bones.**

While not only supporting the body and protecting the systems with a "suit of armor," bones provide movement, along with muscles that allow for walking, sitting, and all movements of the body, both gross and fine. In addition, the bone cells constantly destroy and replace themselves, requiring calcium and phosphorus obtained from other parts of body. This lends to a structural repair and replacement as we age, to maintain our own infrastructure. The skeletal system also is crucial to red blood cell formation.

**There are three types of muscle tissue, and all perform specific functions in the body: voluntary striped muscle, involuntary smooth muscle, and heart muscle.** Muscles are not just our biceps or quadriceps, not just what we outwardly see. They are involved with breathing (the diaphragm), the heart's pumping (cardiac muscle) as well as digestion through peristalsis of the esophagus, small, and large intestine.

Structures that comprise this system, besides the muscle tissue, include tendons. Tendons attach muscles to bones. This system provides movement of all extremities, stabilizing posture and ability to stand upright, allows facial expressions, the generation of heat, and assists in metabolism. As the skeletal and muscular systems are so related in their structure and function, they are often assessed together or referred to as the "Musculoskeletal System."

*The Muscular System:*

**Muscles are not just the outward structures**, such as the biceps in the arms or quadriceps in the legs, that we exercise at the gym to strengthen, define, and tone. Inwardly, for example, they are responsible for breathing (the diaphragm) and movement or flow of body materials such as blood, lymph, food, stool, and sperm.

**Muscles enable body motion** and mobility when working with bones and joints. Stability and posture require skeletal muscles, such as holding the head upright by continual contractions of the neck muscles.

**Elimination** is regulated by constant contraction of smooth muscles in organ **sphincters** to stop outflow of urine or feces, for example.

Muscles, mostly **skeletal muscles, generate heat by their con-traction (thermogenesis)**, and if one shivers from feeling cold, these involuntary contractions increase heat production in the body. Because muscles are vascular, requiring oxygen and pro-ducing heat, the body's natural metabolism is increased due to the energy required to maintain their nutrition and function. That is why **skeletal muscles, even at rest, use and expend more calories than all other tissues.**

Muscles perform these functions through their ability to con-tract (by shortening muscle fibers) and extend (by lengthening fibers) to allow movement, as well as returning to their original state when not in use (contractility, extensibility, and elastic-ity, respectively). Muscles are all nourished by blood (they are vascular).

**In addition, nervous tissue is present in muscles.** This allows muscles to react, voluntary or involuntarily, to a stimulus and transmit these nerve signals through muscle tissue for continued instructions for movements.

**There are three types of muscles,** and each type is categorized by its structure and function. Primarily function only will be addressed. However, microscopic structure is important in how they are named.

**Cardiac muscle** is found only in the heart. It is "striated" be-cause the individual muscle fibers appear striped, like a zebra. It functions involuntary (cannot be controlled) and allows the heart to beat on its own (auto-rhythmicity).

**Smooth muscle** is also involuntary, but because it lacks

stripes, it is classified as smooth (non-striated). It is found inside the walls of unfilled, hollow, space-containing structures (such as blood vessels, airways, urinary bladder, intestines, for example) to transport materials, such as blood cells and plasma, oxygen, urine, nutrients, and waste. One example of involuntary muscular movement occurs in the esophagus via peristalsis. **Peristalsis is a muscular force present in various organs. It functions by alternating muscular contraction with relaxation** of muscles to push food, for example, forward, in a "wavelike" movement, from the back of the throat (pharynx) into the stomach. We have no external or conscious power regarding the movement of the food after swallowing, and it is completely involuntary.

However, when discussing muscles of the musculoskeletal system, it is a third type of muscles that is significant to this grouping of the two systems. These are the **skeletal muscles. They are voluntary** in how they function (under our conscious control) and striated. Attached to bones via tendons, these muscles contract and relax at our will and conscious command to provide movement by exerting their force on bones. One end of the muscle (the head) is attached to an immobile structure (the origin). The other end (the insertion) is attached to the bone that permits movement. The bulk of the muscle between these two ends is the belly of the muscle. **In all, there are more than 600 individually named and recognized skeletal muscles that comprise this system besides the connective tissue,** tendons, which form from and attach most muscles to the bones. Both bones and tendons are named and classified according to the body part where they are located.

*The Skeletal System:*

**There are 206 bones that are identified in the human body and all fall within one of two classifications: the axial skeleton or appendicular skeleton. The axial skeletal group pertains to the trunk of the body and totals 80 bones. It includes all bones that are midline in the body** including the skull and facial bones (22 bones), the hyoid bone near the throat (1), vertebral column (26), ribs (24), sternum (breastbone) (1), and various bones in the ear (6).

**The appendicular skeleton class** is comprised of all the bones in the limbs as well as the bones that connect the limbs to the axial skeleton. This includes the pectoral girdles (4 bones), which connect the arms to the trunk and upper extremities, including the upper arm bone (humerus) to fingers (60), as well as the pelvic girdle (2), which connects the legs to the trunk and the lower extremities from the thigh bone (femur) to the toes (60).

These bones are then categorized based upon structure and function, which is not detailed here. Generally, however, they are classified according to their shape, which include long bones, short bones, flat bones, and irregular bones. Each type provides structural and functional characteristics.

In addition to bones, also associated with this system is the **connective tissue** which binds or facilitates movement and provides connections between bones, and includes **cartilage and ligaments. Cartilage** is necessary for the smooth and fluid movement between bones. This is basically the padding between bones, providing a gliding surface between the bones. It is attached to the skeletal bones directly. **Ligaments**, another type of connective tissue, greatly differ, a band or rope of tissue connecting bones to bones, or bones to cartilage appearing at bone ends. Ligaments provide movement and stability, and in some cases, limit movement so the joint and bones do not overextend.

**The functions of the skeletal system are vital.** Bones function similar to the framework of a house. They are rigid structures that provide the foundation for muscle attachments to allow movement as well as serving as a scaffold to support and sustain all that makes up the human body. While supporting the body structurally, many bones also protect the internal organs: the skull protects the brain; the ribs protect the heart and lungs, for example. Bones are essential for movement. Although muscular contraction is essential for motion, muscles require an entity upon which to act. Bones, when pulled by muscles, assist and allow physical activity and movement of the body.

**Besides allowing for movement and providing structure, bones also provide other essentials for the body.** The skeleton maintains a mineral reserve of calcium and phosphorus, which is essential for muscle contractions, including cardiac muscle, and nerve conductivity. If blood levels of calcium are low, bone will provide missing calcium to sustain essential and critical body balances. Bones "regenerate" themselves; as they constantly break-down and repair themselves via a process, remodeling, essential in healing fracture injuries.

**Parts of bones (red bone marrow) are responsible for producing red blood cells (erythrocytes) for oxygen delivery, white blood cells (leukocytes) for immune function, and platelets (thrombocytes) for clotting.** Production of blood cells is called hemopoiesis. In addition, other part of bones (yellow bone marrow) are responsible for storage of lipids essential for energy.

*Joints (Articulations):*

Because of muscles and bones, the body moves. **But without joints, the body has no fluid movement.** It would be rigid, stiff and unbending. Joints enable the flowing, smooth, and effortless motion provided by our musculoskeletal system. Additionally, it could not provide all of the vast functions that we utilize in our everyday functions.

Joints (articulations) are comprised of skeletal and muscular structures combined with connective tissue which allows diverse movements so we can bend our knees, touch our thumb to our pinky finger, rotate our arm to throw a ball. Joints are classified according to their structure and function, which will not be addressed here.

# REFERENCES

AARP (2015), *AARP THE MAGAZINE,* Oct/Nov 2015, pp. 48-55

Cooper, D.W. (2011). *Ting and I: A Memoir of Love, Courage, and Devotion.* Denver, CO: Outskirts Press.

Davis, N.J. (2015). *The ABCs of Caregiving, Part 2: Essential Information for You and Your Family.* Bellingham, WA: House of Harmony Press.

DeLaune, S. C., & Ladner, P. K. (1998). *Fundamentals of Nursing Standards & Practice.* Albany: Delmar Publishers.

Doenges, M. F. M., & Geissler, A. C. (2000). *Nursing Care Plans, Guidelines for Individualized Patient Care,* Edition 5. Philadelphia: F.A. Davis Company.

Elkin, M. K., Perry, A. G., & Potter, P. A. (2000). *Nursing Interventions & Clinical Skills,* 2nd Edition. St Louis: Mosby.

Grant, R. (2014). *Compliance and How and Why to Avoid an Audit: A Guide to HIPAA and Other Regulatory Compliance Issues.* Greenlawn, NY: Compliancy Group. Amazon ebook.

Gross, A.G., & Cooper, D.W. (2015) *Solved! Curing Your Medical Insurance Problems.* Denver, CO: Outskirts Press.

Lauber, R. (2015), *The Successful Caregiver's Guide*. North Vancouver, BC, Canada: International Self-Counsel Press, Ltd.

LeBlanc, G. J. (2013) *Managing Alzheimer's and Dementia Behaviors: Common Sense Caregiving,* Amazon Digital Services, LLC.

LeMone, P., & Burke, K. M. (2000). *Medical-Surgical Nursing, Critical Thinking in Client Care*, 2nd Edition. Upper Saddle River, NJ: Prentice Hall Health.

Mace, N.L., & Rabins, P.V., *the 36-Hour Day: A Family Guide to Caring for People Who Have Alzheimer Disease, Related Diseases, and Memory Loss, 5th Edition (2011)*, Johns Hopkins Press. Paperback, hardcover, audio book, and Amazon ebook.

Mamou, M. (2014). *Treating Pressure Ulcers and Chronic Wounds*. Course 3457, CME Resource/Net CE. Amazon ebook.

McVeigh, N. (2015). "Leveraging the Power of Technology to Help with Caregiver Duties," Article in the blog lotsahelpinghands.com.

Pharoah, G. (2004, 2013). *How to Manage Family Illness at Home*. Taunton, Somerset, UK: Amolibros.

Scallan, T. L. (2015). *The Ultimate Compassionate Guide to Caregiving: A Simple Blueprint for Dealing with Today's Healthcare Crisis Combined with Years of Wisdom and Sound Advice*. Pasadena, CA: Best Seller Publishing

Seligman, M.E.P. (2002). *Authentic Happiness: Using the New*

*Positive Psychology to Realize Your Potential for Lasting Fulfillment*. New York: Free Press and Simon & Schuster Digital. Hardcover, paperback, and ebook.

Smeltzer, S. C., & Bare, B. G. (2000). *Brunner & Suddarth's Textbook of Medical Surgical Nursing,* 7th Edition. Philadelphia: Lippincott.

*Taber's Cyclopedic Medical Dictionary*, Edition 18 (1997). Philadelphia, PA: F.A. Davis Company.

Tortora, G. J., & Grabowski, S. R. (1996). *Principles of Anatomy and Physiology*, 8th Edition. New York: Harper Collins College Publishers.

Urden, L. D., Stacey, K. M., & Lough, M. E. (2002). *Thelan's Critical Care Nursing Diagnosis and Management,* 4th Edition. St. Louis: Mosby.

Wilkinson, J. M. (2000). *Nursing Diagnosis Handbook*, 7th Edition. Upper Saddle River, NJ: Prentice Hall Health.

Wilson, B. (2014). *Long Term Care: Everything You Need to Know About Long Term Care Nursing and How to Plan and Pay for Long Term Care Insurance*. BMS Publishing. Amazon ebook.

# WEBSITE SOURCES

American Association of Neurological Surgeons:
www.aans.org

American Cancer Association:
www.cancersocietyofamerica.org

American Cancer Society: www.cancer.org

American Diabetes Association: www.diabetes.org

American Heart Association: www.heart.org

American Kidney Fund: www.kidneyfund.org

American Lung Association: www.lung.org

Cancer Society of America: www.cancersocietyofamerica.org

Colostomy Association: www.colostomyassociation.org

Johns Hopkins Medicine: www.hopkinsmedicine.org

Linus Pauling Institute, Oregon State University:
www.lpi.oregonstate.edu

Mayo Clinic: www.mayoclinic.org

MedicineNet.com: www.medicinenet.com

National Cancer Institute: www.cancer.gov

National Center for Biotechnology Information:
www.ncbi.nlm.hih.gov

National Institute of Diabetes and Digestion and Kidney
Disease: www.niddk.nih.gov

National Institute of Neurological Diseases and Stroke: www.ninds.nih.gov

National Parkinson's Foundation: www.parkinsons.org

National Pressure Ulcer Advisory Panel (NPUAP): www.npuap.org

Parkinson's Disease Foundation: www.pdf.org

University of California, San Francisco: www.ucsfhealth.org

United Ostomy Association of America: www.ostomy.org

World Heart Federation: www.heart.org

# APPENDIX 1
# FIVE TIPS FOR EMPOWERED CAREGIVERS

Eboni Green, PhD, RN
Co-Founder of Caregiver Support Services
www.caregiversupportservices.org

Caregivers who are worried, experiencing depression and anxiety will unfortunately experience burnout long-term. In fact, our system cannot afford to lose a single caregiver because they are burned out. Because caring for your loved one can be extremely stressful, I hope that you will use the following tips to care for yourself as you care for your loved one:

**Let go of tasks that you do not need to perform.** This means that sometimes you will need to delegate and let go of tasks that you do not need to perform personally. Perhaps your home will not be as clean as you would like sometimes; in the long run, the cleanliness of your home does not matter. When you delegate, it is important to let the other person complete the task in his or her own time. Remember that you cannot determine someone else's pace, but you can control your response. You can either give the person space to flourish or overshadow his or her important roles by holding on to everything. Your goal is to make sure your loved one is cared for and loved.

**Include others who will assist you.** If you have family and friends on whom you can call for support, it is important to do so. Even if you do not have extended family nearby or do not get along with your own family, you can still build a network of friends who can help in the care of your loved ones; some of them may even become your greatest supporters.

**Celebrate successes along the way.** On occasions where you are successful in reaching a goal, no matter how incremental, you should stop and celebrate. I find that sometimes caregivers minimize the successes that occur in their day. It is important to focus on what is going well if you want to be healthy over the long term.

**Take time out for yourself.** When possible, try to schedule time to do things that are important to you. It is important to make sure that you keep interests outside of your caregiving. When you take time out for yourself, it should be for something that you would not need to do or learn as a part of caring for your loved one.

**Be empowered!** The term *empowerment* is defined as the ability to engage in and execute behaviors for successful caregiving. It is a significant force that may assist you with the tasks associated with caring for a loved one. In fact, once you are empowered, you are better able to help your loved one live life with greater fulfillment. When you are empowered, you are also more inclined to reflect on the many rewards gained by the new sense of purpose resulting from providing care for your loved one.

# APPENDIX 2
# CUSTODIAL CARE AT HOME

A good fraction of the work that needs to be done in caring for a patient in the home is "custodial," the kind of care that might be needed for a healthy baby, rather than "nursing," the kind of care that requires the training that nurses undergo that makes them medical professionals. This appendix is based on a summary of a book that provides excellent instruction in the elements of custodial home care. We strongly advise caregivers to obtain it.

In 2015, Tena L Scallan published her excellent *The Ultimate Compassionate Guide to Caregiving: A Simple Blueprint for Dealing with Today's Healthcare Crisis Combined with Years of Wisdom and Sound Advice*, filled with valuable advice, based on her decades of experience running an agency providing care at home. It has been available as a Kindle ebook for $2.99 and as a 407-page paperback for $14.30. She notes that 1 in 8 Americans are 65 or older, and often children end up taking care of their parents and even their grandparents at a time when both husband and wife may well have jobs outside the home.

**Scallan sees the need for practical advice for caregivers, and her book provides it,** centering on what needs to be done and how to do it, rather than on how to manage it. It makes an excellent companion to our own book.

Scallan starts her book with a set of "absolutes for giving patient care"–never argue, instead agree; don't try to reason, instead divert; don't shame them, instead distract; don't lecture, instead reassure; don't say "remember," instead reminisce; don't say "I told you," instead repeat it; don't say "you can't," instead do what you can; don't command/demand, instead ask/model; don't condescend, instead encourage/praise; don't force, instead reinforce.

Scallan lists these principles of care: safety for yourself and your patient; privacy; dignity; communication, explaining everything as you go along; independence; infection control; being a good listener; being trustworthy; dependability; anger management; managing your own emotions.

Scallan's fine book has the following chapters:

- Communication
- Hygiene and Personal Care
- Medication
- Patient Care Records
- Vital Signs
- Caring and Maintaining a Healthy Environment
- Nutrition
- Body Mechanics and Transferring
- Infection Control
- Safety
- Medical Emergencies
- Emotions
- Legalities
- Insurance
- Expenses

- Informational Documentation Planner
- Resource Guide
- Glossary

We will summarize Scallan's advice, chapter by chapter. When our patient was paraplegic, needing the care provided by a home health aide rather than by a nursing staff, this book would have been exactly what was needed. In several cases, we employed aides who were experienced but lacked formal training, and the insurance company required that we have a nurse certify that they were able to perform the necessary care-giving activities. Having this book available for their instruction would have been a blessing. Much of the care Scallan describes is needed by patients who are receiving skilled nursing care as well.

## Communication

Communication is more than speaking and listening, Scallan notes. Caregivers must give considerable thought to how they are going to present their message to their patients. Getting to know your patient helps. Speaking loudly and slowly and face-to-face is also advisable. Maintain eye contact; ask questions to be sure that the messages are being understood.

Although the patients are often as dependent as children, usually their mental abilities are much greater, so it's important not to be patronizing, not to talk down to them. Empathize with their loss of control over familiar aspects of their lives. Keep it as simple as practical, changing the subject if you note frustration. Realize memory may not be as good as at once was.

## Hygiene and Personal Care

There can be a variety of reasons why the patient may be unable to perform many of the usual tasks for personal hygiene. The caregiver has got to supply these, with patience and consideration, maintaining the dignity of the patient. Scallan gives detailed instructions here for mouth care, bathing, back rubs, manicures and pedicures, hair care, shaving, glasses and contact lenses, hearing aids, dressing and undressing, and adult diapers and associated skin care.

## Medication

Medications include chemicals that require a doctor's prescription and others that are available without one, "over-the-counter (OTC)" medications. Scallan emphasizes the need to follow the medical instructions scrupulously, including the amounts, the timing, the routes of supplying, careful medical record keeping, expiration dates, warnings, patient reactions to the meds.

In boldface capital letters Scallan issues the following alert however:

**MEDICATION ADMINISTRATION—MUST BE DONE BY A FAMILY MEMBER, LICENSED HEALTH CARE PROVIDER OR NURSE. CAREGIVERS CAN ONLY ASSIST WITH MEDICATIONS ALREADY PREPARED BY THE FAMILY MEMBER, HEALTHCARE PROVIDER OR NURSE. HOWEVER, A NURSE MAY BE REQUIRED IF THE PERSON RECEIVING CARE IS UNABLE TO TAKE THEIR MEDICATION WITHOUT ASSISTANCE.**

This warning is for practical and legal reasons, and it is one of the ways in which custodial care is distinguished from skilled nursing care. Tips are provided for the healthcare workers for the administration of the medications already prescribed and prepared. Eye, ear, and nose drops need careful techniques, too, given by Scallan. All medications should be recorded: time, date, medication, dose, how given, and the caregiver initials.

## Patient Care Records

As Scallan notes, "every patient has a care record. This is a permanent written record containing confidential information that serves many purposes:" documentation of the work done, progress, communication among caregivers, basis for evaluating success of the plan, making available information as history for later examination, providing a basis for examining billing.

Detailed guidelines for head-to-toe examination are given. These include observation of appearances and of performance. The ability to perform the routine Activities of Daily Living is noted, as well as the need for assistive equipment.

## Vital Signs

The following are defined in Scallan's section on vital signs: temperature, fever, thermometer, pulse, respiration, blood pressure; the normal ranges for many of these are given, along with the materials and methods used in measurement. Helpfully, the values of some of these measurements that would necessitate contacting the doctor's office are listed. These include temperature, pulse rate, blood pressure, and respiration rate. Scallan emphasizes the necessity of care and cleanliness in taking the patient's vital signs.

## Caring and Maintaining a Healthy Environment

To prevent chemical contamination and to help reduce the risk of infection, the home itself must be kept clean. A wide variety of cleaning supplies will be required. Both disinfecting and cleaning solutions must be employed. The kitchen and dishes and silverware must be kept scrupulously clean. Changing the bed linens while the bed is occupied requires special technique. Laundry can present a challenge. Advice is presented for cleaning urine and fecal stains.

## Nutrition

For home care given by family and home care aides, nutrition will be much the same as done for the family routinely, unless special circumstances apply. Scallan provides valuable information, summarizing much dietary/nutritional material.

Certain handicaps, such as blindness or difficulty with using the hands or arms, will require special feeding approaches.

During periods of skilled nursing care, everything that is ingested will be determined in conjunction with the medical team.

## Body Mechanics and Transferring

Moving the patient, even moving the equipment associated with patient care, is done more safely if attention is given to technique. Scallan gives tips for exercises by the patient as well as step-by-step instructions for proper handling of the patient during movement from one area to another, such as from bed to floor or from chair to standing up. Back injuries are endemic in the caregiving professions, so proper technique, good body mechanics, is essential.

Bedridden patients require frequent movement to prevent bed-sores and promote independence.

A wide variety of assistive devices is available, and their use is well described here.

### Infection Control

Germs are everywhere, including your body, your clothes, your home, household surfaces, *etc*. Cleanliness is the first-line of defense, especially hand washing. In some cases, gloves and face masks may be required.

### Safety

Scallan focuses on "how to reduce your chances of becoming a crime victim." She includes various forms of physical attack and scams.

### Medical Emergencies

Scallan provides a strong disclaimer at the beginning of this section, as dealing with medical emergencies presents risk to the caregiver as well as to the patient. No attempt will be made here to summarize her information, for the same reasons.

### Emotions

Emotions have developed partly to enhance our survival chances: fear, need, loneliness, even love play roles. Decision making is aided and harmed by emotions; you must care, but not be paralyzed with fear. Emotions help us set boundaries between ourselves and others, with both positive and negative impacts. Emotions assist our communications. We need both happiness and occasional sadness to feel alive. They help us bond with others.

Managing negative emotions can be aided by identifying them clearly and then determining whether the feeling is healthful. If not, ask what would help. In communicating them: don't be dramatic, nor let them build up, present them succinctly, avoiding placing blame, and if possible try to diffuse confrontation by offering the other person the opportunity to "safe face," to back down gracefully. Disappointment arises when reality confronts illusions. Bitterness is extreme disappointment. The patient's expectations may have been quite unrealistic, however, as may have been the caregiver's. Discouragement is self-defeating, though understandable.

Positive emotions include hope, love, affection, friendliness, resiliency, forgiveness, and understanding. Help the patient to focus on these, if possible.

Sometimes, laughter is the best medicine.

## Legalities

Useful legal documents include: letter of instruction, living will, power of attorney, reverse mortgage, long-term care insurance policy, do not resuscitate (DNR) order...and we end this list to quote Scallan, as we agree with her concern, "Inconsistent application of DNR orders means some patients get less-than-optimal care once providers are aware of the presence of a

DNR order. There still needs to be more study on this issue, but some health-care providers will even disregard basic care to patients with DNR orders. Because of these issues, for anything other than a terminal diagnosis—like cancer or some end-stage chronic conditions—getting a DNR order may not be the right decision." Neither of our two home-bound patients had a DNR order.

## Insurance

Common options for medical insurance include Medicare Part A, which is hospital insurance; Medicare Part B, which is insurance for most other medical services, Medicare Part C, sometimes called Medicare Advantage, which allows you to receive your care through a provider organization; and Medicare Part D, prescription drug coverage. We discuss these elsewhere in our book. Besides these options there are various private insurance plans, including those provided by businesses and other organizations. Disability insurance can be viewed as a form of medical insurance. Related forms of compensation include Veterans' benefits and Workman's Compensation. Scallan helpfully provides much detail on all of these.

## Expenses

Scallan gives extended advice on managing money during retirement.

## Informational Documentation Planner

Scallan presents a detailed form that goes into specifics on recording essentials related to: emergency information, important contact numbers, healthcare contacts, family and friends, services, and numbers and access codes, medical history, family genealogy, bank accounts, foreign bank accounts, automatic bill paying, personal loans, savings certificates, savings bonds, stock certificates, safe-deposit boxes, cash on hand, home safe, credit union, pension, retirement account, will, trust, living will, durable power of attorney, durable power of attorney for medical care, letter of instruction, religious affiliation, funeral instructions, donor arrangements, autopsy arrangements, cemetery plot, Social Security information, military discharge papers, income tax filings, passport, driver's license, birth certificate, adoption papers, naturalization papers, marriage license, divorce decree, credit cards, Medicare/Medicaid, health insurance policies, long-term care insurance policy, life insurance policy, disability insurance policy, homeowners insurance policy, auto/vehicle insurance policies, vehicle ownership, real estate ownership, school records, employment history, pet history, with some detailed sub-entries for all of these.

**Resource Guide**

Scallan gives the address and phone numbers and a brief description for each of the following:

- Administration on Aging
- Aging Network Services
- American Association of Homes for the Aging
- American Association of Retired Persons (AARP)
- American Geriatrics Society
- American Health Care Association
- American Society on Aging

- B'nai B'rith International
- Catholic Charities
- Catholic Golden Age
- Children of Aging Parents
- Disabled American Veterans
- Episcopal Society for Ministry to the Aging
- Foundation for Hospice and Home Care
- Gray Panthers
- National Association for Home Care
- National Association of Area Agencies on Aging
- National Association of State Units on Aging
- National Council on the Aging
- National Hispanic Council on Aging
- National Hospice Association
- National Institute on Aging
- National Shut-in Society
- Older Women's League
- U.S. Office of Disease Prevention and Health Promotion
- United Way of America
- Veterans Administration
- Volunteers of America

Scallan follows this with similar information on more organizations, categorized by their specific areas of concern: Alzheimer's disease, arthritis, cancer, caregiving, dental health, diabetes, foot care, health, hearing impairment, high blood pressure, housing/long-term care, incontinence, legal issues, medications, nutrition, osteoporosis, safety, stress, stroke, vision. Next, she gives addresses and telephone numbers for the state offices of aging, from Alabama to Wyoming.

The last third of Scallan's *The Ultimate Compassionate Guide to Caregiving* is over one-hundred pages of Glossary, giving in-depth definitions of relevant terms.

To repeat, this is an extraordinarily fine book, which makes a fine companion to ours. Scallan's is directed primarily toward how to **provide custodial care,** generally given by those who are not nurses, and ours deals primarily with **managing nursing care.** In the home situation, custodial care may be being supplied by the family even as nursing care is being supplied by nurses, so that both books may be of use.

# APPENDIX 3
# ACTS OF KINDNESS TOWARD CAREGIVERS

Ideas for acts of kindness toward caregivers, adapted from a list presented by Meghan Bogardus in *AARP THE MAGAZINE*, OCT/NOV 2015, pp. 56-58:

- Bring a low-maintenance houseplant
- Take in the mail
- Shovel snow from the driveway and walkway
- Go grocery shopping
- Arrange a play date for the kids
- Gas up the car
- Do a load of laundry
- Take the kids to a movie
- Send flowers
- Sing some songs
- Play a board game
- Go out for coffee
- Visit with a sweet pet
- Treat to a spa or exercise class
- Take the dog for a walk
- Bring packages to the post office
- Give a massage
- Water the flowers
- Do the dishes
- Bring a movie to watch together
- Return library books

- Volunteer to wait for a service provider
- Mow the lawn
- Help compose a letter
- Wash the car
- Treat to a housecleaning visit
- Donate vacation days
- Replace missing buttons
- Clean the gutters
- Bring coffee or tea
- Drive the kids
- Replace the batteries in smoke detectors
- Tell her how much she's appreciated
- Send a thinking-of-you card
- Take to a comedy club
- Braid her hair
- Cut some extra slack
- Make a CD
- Take out the trash
- Give a blank journal
- Let vent
- Arrange for home organizer
- Help with the garden
- Tell a joke
- Bring over a nice bottle of wine
- Change the oil
- Complain less
- Knit a sweater
- Do an item on the to-do list
- Bring a favorite book
- Bring Sunday paper
- Arrange yoga session
- Do DVD workout together

- Make photo album together
- Hire a message therapist
- Register them with the fancy food club
- Hire a geek to help
- Give luxury-travel magazine
- Meditate together
- Take a portrait with a camera
- Fix a leaky faucet
- Buy an e-reader
- Pick up the dry cleaning
- Rake the leaves
- Play cards
- Hire a personal shopper
- Give a gift card to favorite restaurant
- Help write a thank-you note
- Mail a care package
- Attend the meeting and take notes
- Set up a meditation appointment
- Send a skywriter message
- Donate a casserole
- Bake cookies
- Help decorate for the holidays
- Decorate the walkway
- Pay a compliment
- Set up bird feeder
- Work her shift
- Drop off a prescription
- Create a relaxing space in the home
- Paint a picture
- Write a poem
- Give scented oil
- Assist child with college application
- Take old clothes to the thrift store

# APPENDIX 4
# THE SUCCESSFUL CAREGIVER'S GUIDE

This excellent book by Canadian writer Rick Lauber (2015) shares the lessons he and his two sisters learned while caring for and obtaining care for their mother (Parkinson's) and their father (Alzheimer's). His book is directed not only to teaching how to provide and obtain care for loved ones, in his case his parents, but also how to assure that the caregiver takes adequate care of himself. The book is particularly good on the psycho-social aspects of caregiving for one's ill parents.

Here is the table of contents:

Chapter 1: Defining Caregiving
   1. The Different Types of Caregivers
   2. What Type of Caregiver Are You?
Worksheet 1: Caregiving Self-Analysis
Worksheet 2: Your Circle of Caregiving

Chapter 2: Caring from a Distance
   1. The Challenges of Long-Distance Caregiving
   2. What to Do When You Get There
   3. Find the Necessary Information and Documents
   4. Check the Safety of Your Parents' Home
   5. Respect the Decision That Not Everyone Wants to Relocate
   6. Emotional Distance
Worksheet 3: Home Safety Checklist

Lauber offers a set of forms in Word or PDF format to help you keep track of caregiving needs, via this URL

www.self-counsel.com/updates/successfulcaregiver/15kit.htm

For Example, here is Worksheet 1:

**Worksheet 1**
**Caregiving Self-Analysis**

Self-evaluation is crucial to caregivers. While you will be presented with many new responsibilities and challenges, you must know what you can do and the extent of your own personal limits.

Answer the following questions as honestly as you can. Addressing these issues sooner rather than later will help you identify your own strengths and weaknesses, which will be beneficial to you as a caregiver. Share these questions (and your answers, if you feel comfortable) with your siblings and delegate your roles appropriately.

1. What can you do as a caregiver?
2. How do you feel about becoming and acting as a caregiver?
3. What would you identify as your characteristic strengths and weaknesses?
4. Who will help you with your caregiving responsibilities? (Identify what others can do.)
5. Beyond your immediate circle of contacts, where will you look for additional help?
6. Can you work easily with others or do you prefer to work independently?

7. Are you flexible with your own schedule?
8. What negative issues do you foresee with serving as a caregiver?
9. How will you respond to or counteract these negative issues?
10. Where will you seek respite for your loved one?
11. Where will you seek respite for yourself?
12. List three additional ideas for personal coping and caring mechanisms. (These will be new areas of interest to you that you could try in the future.)
13. How much personal respite time will you give yourself?
14. What do you want to achieve as a caregiver?
15. Are you hesitant or reluctant to serve as a caregiver? If so, why?
16. How much will this hesitation interfere with your caregiving duties?
17. Will you be able to perform certain tasks or do you need to assign them to others?
18. Can you honestly look at yourself in the mirror and say, "I am doing the best job I can as a caregiver"?
19. Do you have any regrets about serving as a caregiver? If so, what are your regrets and how can you resolve them?
20. Where can you learn more about your loved one's medical condition and prognosis?
21. What other personal or professional demands, besides caregiving, exist for you?
22. How will you know you have done your best being a caregiver?
23. Are you an optimist or a pessimist? (Note that optimists will have an easier time and might be better caregivers.)

# APPENDIX 5
# NURSING CARE PLAN EXAMPLE

The following is an actual care plan submitted by this writer [DRB] while in nursing school. It is provided to illustrate nursing care plans. Some information has been altered or deleted for patient confidentially. [Bracketed material added editorially here.]

**Name:** Diane Beggin **Date:** 04-11-02 **Client**: E.J. **MedDx:** Syncopal Episodes, Acute Renal Failure, Possible Pneumonia

**Nsg Dx:** Impaired Gas Exchange related to decreased functioning lung tissue, chemotherapeutic agents, decreased immune response and congestion secondary to recent thoracotomy of mesothelioma (diagnosed in 10/2001), chemotherapy Gemcitabine and Cisplatin.

**Defining Characteristics:** As Evidenced By—increased respiration rate typically above 20 up to 28-34 breaths per minute (normal = 16-20) noted intermittently but usually upon restlessness or exertion at bedside; audible breath sounds without auscultation indicative of fluid congestion in lungs; ineffective, unproductive cough with retained secretions; decreased oxygen saturation of 92% on 2L oxygen via nasal cannula (normal with room air is 96% plus). Lab values: hyper- to hypocapnia [high to low levels of carbon dioxide in the blood] (20-42mmHg when normal limits are between 22-29mmHg); hypoxemia [low levels of oxygen in the blood] (74 when normal is between 80-100); decreased hemoglobin (9-10g/100mL when normal is between 13.5-17g/100mL), decreased hematocrit (28-31% when normal is 41-53%); decreased erythrocytes (3.6-3.7million/mm3 when normal is 4.7-6.1million/mm3). Mental status: restless intermittently; confusion "Is WWI over?" WWII? "What war is going on now?" "Am I still at City Hospital?" (When actually that hospital was in a different state in a different part of the country.)

**Outcome:** Client will have increased gas exchange within four days as evidenced by: decreased confusion and restlessness; increased level of consciousness; decreased dyspnea at rest and upon exertion in 24 hours or less; decrease in adventitious [unusual, non-normal] breath sounds especially those heard without auscultation; ABGs with normal ranges; increased sputum to relieve congestion.

**Interventions [I] & Rationales [R]:**

1) **I:** Assess lungs every 2 hours minimum or upon changes. Assess for unauscultated [not sensed by a stethoscope] audible and auscultated congestion. Note type and presence of adventitious lung sounds as well if diminished. (Assessed with wheezes bilaterally, crackles especially to left base, diminished on right and unknown to what extent lung was dissected). Note location.

   **R:** Frequent assessment lends to knowledge of progressing or resolving problems and provides increased time to act. Noting specifics provides baseline for self and others to use for comparison in evaluation of treatment.

**2) I:** Assess rate and quality of respirations every 2 hours. Look for increases in signs of dyspnea such as nasal flaring, shallow respirations, tachypnea, increased confusion and restlessness, decrease in capillary refill (currently normal) and decreased peripheral pulses (present currently).

**R:** All are additional signs of lack of oxygen via gas exchange. Some provide details of progression to other systems such as the periphery if changes occur.

**3) I:** Monitor neurological functions every 2 hours. Establish baseline for level of consciousness, papillary response, response to sensation, command response. Provide simple commands in which he can follow. Orientate as necessary.

**R:** After initial assessment, baseline provides gauge upon which to further assess. Level of consciousness is primary indicator. Already has decreased function to time and place. Can easily lose track of times especially with currently prescribed medications. Helps to provide recognition to surroundings and focus.

**4) I:** Ensure oxygen is provided as ordered. Check position of cannula and skin to ensure no breakdown. Collaborate with respiratory therapy to ensure treatments are completed as ordered. Follow up on arterial blood gas orders.

**R:** With decreased oxygen to tissues, integrity of skin can diminish, increasing risk for infection. Ensures proper placement to ensure therapeutic measure. Ensures treatments are received timely and do not interfere with other diagnostic tests or treatments. Values essential to provide meaningful and therapeutic treatments.

5) **I:** Elevate head of bed to roughly semi-Fowler's position or as is comfortable for client. Ensure proper precaution (use of pillows, flexion at knee, *etc.*) to decrease shearing forces especially with lack of energy to prop self up and prevent sliding.

**R:** Provides increased oxygenation by decreasing pressure on diaphragm and result in ease of breathing. Position helps with problems with hypoxia and hypoxemia.

6) **I:** When conscious and alert, encourage deep breathing. Find ways to enhance client participation (for example, washing feet makes him more alert; smiling at him evokes the same response). At those times, instruct him to deep breathe and mime it for him. Provide splinting for his coughing as he had decreased energy and unable to do it himself.

**R:** Client is cooperative. When alert, encouraging and taking deep breaths with him may decrease avoidance or increase mimic activity. Due to confusion, splint abdomen for him to illustrate. Continue to do so when can each time, doing these exercises until he can accomplish them for himself.

7) **I:** Ensure suction equipment is accessible.

**R:** Provides readiness in negative circumstances.

**8) I:** Encourage fluids as appropriate. Client has no IV except for pharmacological treatment and is on a renal diet. For comfort, provide mouth care every 2 hours if not more.

**R:** Without fluids mouth becomes very dry. Also on antibiotics with increased risk for thrush increased with leukocytopenia [a decrease in the white blood cells]. Mouth care provides freshness, comfort, hygiene, and opportunity for assessment.

# EXHIBIT LISTING

EXHIBIT #1:   SHIFT SCHEDULE

EXHIBIT #2A:  PHYSICIAN'S ORDERS—DAILY & PRN
MEDICATIONS

EXHIBIT #2B:  PHYSICIAN'S ORDERS—EQUIPMENT &
TREATMENTS

EXHIBIT #3:   EMERGENCY PLAN

EXHIBIT #4:   REFERENCE INFORMATION & CONTACTS

EXHIBIT #5A:  MONTHLY NURSING TREATMENT
FORM—PAGE 1

EXHIBIT #5B:  MONTHLY NURSING TREATMENT
FORM—PAGE 3

EXHIBIT #6A:  DAILY MEDICATION ADMINISTRATION
RECORD—PAGE 1

EXHIBIT #6B:  PRN MEDICATION ADMINISTRATION
RECORD—PAGE 6

EXHIBIT #7A:  NURSING REVIEW / ASSESSMENT
FORM—PAGE 1

# EXHIBIT #1:
# SHIFT SCHEDULE

TENTATIVE SCHEDULE FOR **AUGUST 2015**    [MAY 31]

|    |     |         |         |           | O/N [10P-8A, x Th] |
|----|-----|---------|---------|-----------|--------------------|
| 01 | SAT | 8A-4P EP |        | 4P-10P MB | SC |
| 02 | SUN | 8A-4P BT |        | 4P-10P CP | DO |
|    |     |         |         |           |    |
| 03 | MON | 8A-4P MW |        | 4P-10P CP | AP |
| 04 | TUE | 8A-2P DO |        | 2P-10P MB | BT |
| 05 | WED | 8A-4P MW |        | 4P-10P CP | AP |
| 06 | THU | 8A-1P DO | 1P-6P KK | 6P-11P BT | AP(11) |
| 07 | FRI | 8A-1P DO |        | 1P-10P KK | BT |
| 08 | SAT | 8A-4P DB |        | 4P-10P HG | AP |
| 09 | SUN | 8A-4P BT |        | 4P-10P CP | DO |
|    |     |         |         |           |    |
| 10 | MON | 8A-4P MW |        | 4P-10P CP | AP |
| 11 | TUE | 8A-2P MW |        | 2P-10P MB | BT |
| 12 | WED | 8A-4P MW |        | 4P-10P CP | AP |
| 13 | THU | 8A-1P DO | 1P-6P KK | 6P-11P BT | AP(11) |
| 14 | FRI | 8A-1P DO |        | 1P-10P KK | BT |
| 15 | SAT | 8A-4P EP |        | 4P-10P MB | SC |
| 16 | SUN | 8A-4P BT |        | 4P-10P CP | DO |
|    |     |         |         |           |    |
| 17 | MON | 8A-4P MW |        | 4P-10P CP | AP |
| 18 | TUE | 8A-2P DO |        | 2P-10P MB | BT |
| 19 | WED | 8A-4P MW |        | 4P-10P CP | AP |
| 20 | THU | 8A-1P DO | 1P-6P KK | 6P-11P BT | AP(11) |
| 21 | FRI | 8A-1P DO |        | 1P-10P KK | BT |
| 22 | SAT | 8A-4P DB |        | 4P-10P HG | AP |
| 23 | SUN | 8A-4P BT |        | 4P-10P CP | DO |
|    |     |         |         |           |    |
| 24 | MON | 8A-4P MW |        | 4P-10P CP | AP |
| 25 | TUE | 8A-2P MW |        | 2P-10P MB | BT |
| 26 | WED | 8A-4P MW |        | 4P-10P CP | AP |
| 27 | THU | 8A-1P DO | 1P-6P KK | 6P-11P BT | AP(11) |
| 28 | FRI | 8A-1P DO |        | 1P-10P KK | BT |
| 29 | SAT | 8A-4P EP |        | 4P-10P MB | SC |
| 30 | SUN | 8A-4P BT |        | 4P-10P CP | DO |
|    |     |         |         |           |    |
| 31 | MON | 8A-4P MW |        | 4P-10P CP | AP |

**PHONE NUMBERS**
DB = Diane Beggin (xxx) xxx-xxxx
MB = Melissa xxxx   etc.

# EXHIBIT #2A:
# PHYSICIAN'S ORDERS—DAILY & PRN MEDICATIONS—PAGE 1

## PHYSICIAN'S ORDERS
### DAILY & PRN MEDICATIONS (page 1 of 2)

**Client Information:**

Name: Patient Name    DOB: 10/06/1946    Age: 68
Address: 389 Bluejay Drive, Hudson, NY 12621
Telephone: 807.555.2481
Allergies: Erythromycin

**Medical Background & History:**

Diagnosis: MS End Stage; s/p R Breast Mastectomy without nodal involveme

Prognosis: Poor - __X__    Guarded: _____    Fair - _____    Good - _____

Factors: Tracheostomy w/ventilator & $O_2$ support; Peg tube; Quadraplegic w/severe bilateral contractures; Pain

**Medication Administration: Daily**

| Routine | Dosage | Frequency | Route |
|---|---|---|---|
| Liquid Nutrition | 250mL | 4 daily | GT |
| Carafate (sucralfate) | 1gm | q6h | GT |
| Prozac (fluoxetine HCl) | 20mg | TID | GT |
| Baclofen (lioresal) | 40mg total | TID | GT / 20mg AM, 10mg af 10mg evening |
| Norvasc (amlodipine besylate) | 2.5mg | BID | GT |
| * Sodium | 1gm | BID | GT |
| Iron supplement | 28mg | daily | GT |
| Calcium supplement | 600mg | daily | GT |
| K-Elixer | 40mEq | daily | GT |
| Vitamin B12 | 1000mcg | daily | GT |
| Magnesium Oxide | 240-400mg | daily | GT |
| Aspirin | 81mg | daily | GT |
| Ducolax Suppository | i | MWF | rectal |
| Senokot | ii | SunTTh | GT |
| Ativan (lorazepam) | 2mg | HS | GT |
| Miralax | ≤17gm | per regime | GT |

# EXHIBIT #2A:
# PHYSICIAN'S ORDERS—DAILY & PRN
# MEDICATIONS—PAGE 2

## PHYSICIAN'S ORDERS
## DAILY & PRN MEDICATIONS (page 2 of 2)

**Client Information:**

Name: Patient Name    DOB: 10/06/1946    Age: 68
Allergies: Erythromycin

**Medication Administration: PRN**

| PRN | Dosage | Frequency | Route |
|---|---|---|---|
| Ativan (lorazepam) | 0.5mg | PRN x1 | GT / for anxiety & repet |
| Halcion (triazolam) | 0.25mg | PRN - HS | GT / for insomnia |
| Morphine Sulfate | 15-30mg | PRN q6h | GT / for pain |
| Lidoderm 5% Transdermal | 0.5-1 patch | PRN | Topical to area of pain; |
| Fleet Glycerin Suppository | "bullet" | PRN | Rectal / for constipation |
| Magnesium Citrate | 5oz | PRN | GT / for constipation |
| Fleet Phosphosoda | 1.5oz | PRN | GT / for constipation |
| Imodium | 20ml | PRN | GT / for diarrhea |
| Sodium Bicarb | 1/4 tsp:60mLH2O | PRN | GT / upset stomach / n |
| Desoximetasone 0.25% | thin layer | PRN - BID | Topical to trach stoma / |
| Nasocort (trimcinolone) | ii sprays | PRN x i | Nasal / for congestion - |
| Benadryl | 12.5mg | PRN | GT / for allergies. |
| Sudafed | 30mg | PRN | GT / for allergies. |
| Liquid Nutrition | ≤250ml | PRN | GT / for hunger |

**Physician Information:**

Name: Frank Ggg, MD
Address: 6250 East Bradley Street, P.O. Box 856-2621, Hudson, NY 12621
Telephone: 807.555.6666    Fax: 807.555.6667

Signature: _____    Date: __

* indicates change from previous orders.        Prepared by: D. Beggin, RN  (09/2015)

# EXHIBIT #2B:
# PHYSICIAN'S ORDERS—
# EQUIPMENT & TREATMENTS—PAGE 1

## PHYSICIAN'S ORDERS
## EQUIPMENT & TREATMENTS (page 1 of 2)

### Client Information:

**Name:**    Patient Name      **DOB:** 10/06/1946    **Age:** 68

**Address:**  389 Bluejay Drive, Hudson, NY 12621

**Telephone:**  807.555.2481

**Allergies:**  Erythromycin

### Medical Background & History:

**Diagnosis:**  MS End Stage; s/p R Breast Mastectomy without nodal involvement

**Prognosis:**  Poor - __X__    Guarded: _____    Fair - _____    Good - _____

**Factors:**  Tracheostomy w/ventilator & $O_2$ support; Peg tube; Quadraplegic w/severe bilateral contractures; Pain

### Routine Orders & Care:

**Activities:**  1) Bedbath - Complete - __X__    Partial Assist - _____

                2) Bedrest - Complete - __X__    Partial - _____    As tolerable - _____

                3) Out of Bed - As tolerable with Full assist & Hoyer Transfer

**Nutrition:**  1) NPO;    2) Complete liquid nutrition w/fiber x 4 bolus feedings daily - 250mL/can, each 250 calories;

                3) Protein supplement 4 scoops daily if not supplied in feeding;

                4) Cranberry juice light 240/mL day;    5) Yogurt 60mL per day;

                6) Fluid intake >2000ml/day;    7) Fluids delivered via peg slow bolus.

**Discipline:**  RN - __X__  / LPN - __X__  for __24__ hours/day  for __7__ days/week

### Equipment:

**Bed:**  Hospital - _____        Air Mattress - __X__

**Mobility:**  Wheelchair - __X__        Hoyer Lift - __X__

**Respiration:**  Ventilator - __X__        Oxygen Concentrator - __X__

                  Ventilator Settings/SIMV;  Tidal Volume/450;  Pressure Support/12;

                  Breath Rate = 10;  PEEP = 3;  Oxygen Concentrator Setting = 3L

# EXHIBIT #2B:
# PHYSICIAN'S ORDERS—EQUIPMENT & TREATMENTS—PAGE 2

---

## PHYSICIAN'S ORDERS
## EQUIPMENT & TREATMENTS (page 2 of 2)

---

**Client Information: Continued**

Name:   Patient Name        DOB: 10/06/1946    Age: 68

---

**Treatments / Nursing Functions:**

### GENERAL NURSING CARE:

Observe Standard Precautions at all times.

Change depends minimum q4h & supplement
   with inserts to maintain skin integrity & hygiene.

Perform breast exam qMonth including
   nodes under axilla.

Turn and position to

Provide PROM to upp
   qShift.

Check air mattress to
   tubing for possi

### RESPIRATORY TREATMENTS & CARE:

Check vent circuit & settings qShift.

Follow trach cuff protocol: 2-10mL to maintain
   tidal volume ~450 using lowest cuff volume.

Provide 35% humidification via trach collar with
   $O_2$ @3L when off vent as needed.

Assess skin under trach ties daily.

Change inner cannula & HME daily.

Change $O_2$ tubing q2Weeks

**Maintain SaO$_2$** >95%
   if SaO$_2$ is <92%.

Suction as required &

**Provide trach** stoma c

**0.9% Nor**mal Sa

Change in-line suctio
   q3days.

Change condensor &

### GASTROINTESTINAL TREATMENT & CARE:

Follow enteral feeding precautions at all times.

Flush peg tube with 100mL $H_2O$ post feedings & med
   admin. Dilute meds in 10mL $H_2O$ minimum.

Perform peg care by cleaning with $H_2O_2$ BID. Apply
   A&D post cleaning & PRN.

Change 60mL bulb s
   admin qMonth &

**Monitor bowel** elimina

**necessa**ry.

**Note PEG tube** is 20F

---

**Physician Information:**

Name:       Frank Ggg , MD
Address:    6250 East Bradley Street, P.O. Box 856-2621, Hudson, NY  12621
Telephone:  807.555.6666        Fax: 807.555.6667

Signature: _____   Date: _____

\* indicates change from previous orders.    Prepared by: D. Beggin, RN  (09/2015)

### PHYSICIAN'S ORDERS—DAILY & PRN MEDICATIONS
### PHYSICIAN'S ORDERS—EQUIPMENT & TREATMENTS

Two sets of physician orders are included here. These are orders given by the doctor to provide nurses with the ability to administer medications and provide ordered care. Orders are defined by whether they are medication based or treatment based. Both order sets must be reviewed and renewed by the physician at regular intervals.

The fields that are the same for both sets of orders are detailed first. These include Client Information, Medical Background & History, Physician Information, and a detail line for in-house tracking.

**"Client Information":** This section provides patient information for the physician. Also included is a listing of all allergies, date of birth, and current age. This information proves vital in prescribing or not prescribing medications, based upon age and what is tolerable for the patient. This field is the same for the medication and equipment orders.

**"Medical Background & History":** A snapshot of the patient's medical history is provided here. Included are the most notable, chronic, or existing conditions for which continuing care is required for the patient, as well as factors that may impact future physician decisions and orders. This field is the same for the medication and equipment orders.

**"Physician Information":** This field indicates the name and contact information of the physician who is renewing the orders.

Provided is a signature and date line. This field, too, is the same for the medication and equipment orders.

**Tracking Line:** There is a line appearing below the physician information on the last page of the forms which we utilize as a means to track changes from one 90-day period to the next. To assist the physician and us, we denote changes from the previously submitted orders versus the present with an asterisk. We also include the nurse who provided the documentation to the physician and the 90-day date. This is done internally for record-keeping and ease in differentiating what, if any, changes were made to the orders from the previous submission.

The sections of the two physician orders that differ from each other pertain only to actual medications and treatments which are necessary for continuing care. **Medication orders** solely list all of the pharmaceutically prescribed and over-the-counter [OTC] medications that this patient receives on a daily basis and medications that may be given [PRN] to her if the need arises. **Treatments and equipment orders** list what is necessary for her continued health that is not a medication. Simply stated, it is a "to-do" list that is essential for her survival.

**"Medication Administration: Daily & PRN":** The fields in these tables document medications that have been newly ordered and/or renewed by the physician. There is a separate table for meds that are given daily ("Routine") and a separate one for medications which are ordered but are only administered if and when necessary according to circumstances ("PRN"). For this patient, most PRN medications address pain and bowel function. A definition for each column within these sections follows:

**"Routine" or "PRN":** Each medication name is listed in the first column under the heading of Routine (or daily) or PRN . When pertinent, brand and generic names are both provided.

**"Dosage":** This specifies the amount to be given at each time: this is not a daily amount.

**"Frequency":** How many times daily medication is administered is provided here. Medical abbreviations are illustrated here but "every 6 hours" for q6h, or "two times a day" for *bid*, *etc.* may be used.

**"Route":** The method by which the medication is administered, or how the patient will receive the med, is noted here. As this patient has a gastric tube and is NPO, any medication that would normally be administered orally is given to her via the tube. Therefore, medications designated "GT" are given in liquid (or crushed in water) through the tube. Other routes are "rectally" for suppositories and "topical" for creams or ointments and the location of the body to which they should be applied. Pertinent notes are also indicated here, for example the reason why a PRN medication may be given such as for pain, constipation, or skin rash.

**"Routine Orders & Care":** It includes activities of daily living, nutritional support, and what discipline is necessary for patient care.

**"Equipment":** This information provides a listing of actual equipment that the patient requires for complete care. Items listed here include furniture, such as hospital beds and wheel chairs, and any other equipment that is essential. Illustrated here, a ventilator is required for the patient. The settings, as determined by the physician are also included.

**"Treatments / Nursing Functions":** These entries compile a detailed, although not complete, list of nursing actions essential and required for the continued care of the patient. They do not include medications. Specific and comprehensive to patient care, equipment, and timing of equipment changes or nursing actions that are physician ordered are noted, and they are arranged by physiological system. Parameters for equipment use, settings, or instructions for replacement are also provided. This does not detail all the necessary treatments which are required, but gives instructions when such equipment changes and treatments are minimally necessary. This provides details for insurance purposes as well.

# EXHIBIT #3:
# EMERGENCY PLAN

## EMERGENCY PLAN (04-2015)

For **ALL** Situations — **IF** Spouse is **NOT** in the residence
Telephone him **ASAP** after patient is stabilized.

> **LOSS OF ELECTRICAL POWER:**

**Immediately** attend to patient and reassure her as numerous alarms will sound.

    A. VENTILATOR: This has its own battery, approximately lasting for 30 minutes. Near the wheelchair in the dining room, there are 2 rectangular grey batteries good for 3 hours each.
       1. Connect vent to the back-up battery.
       2. Reset the alarm by as you would during, for example, a high pressure signal.
       3. The gasoline-powered generator can also be run if needed. Spouse will attend to this.
    B. OXYGEN SUPPLY: The concentrator will stop, therefore $O_2$ supply will stop.
       1. Disconnect $O_2$ tubing from concentrator.
       2. Attach tubing to an $O_2$ cylinder.
       3. Open Cylinder:
          With Wrist Lever: 1) keep lever horizontal; 2) turn to the left (counter-clockwise).
          With Wrench: 1) use second slot; 2) turn to the left (counter-clockwise).
       4. Set Flow Rate at 1LPM
    C. PULSE OXIMETER: This has a battery. Use briefly but frequently.
    D. SUCTION: This has a battery. Use as needed.
    E. LIGHT: Flashlights are available by the front door and in her bedroom.
    F. COMMUNICATION: Cell phones should work, but land lines will not. If spouse is not in the, residence, call him via your cell.
    G. RETURN OF POWER or USE OF GENERATOR: Once power is obtained, be sure to restart $O_2$ concentrator manually, as it doesn't automatically restart and resume.

> **LOSS OF VENTILATOR:**

Reassure patient and disconnect her from vent. She can sustain on HME alone for a short period.

    A. Disconnect vent circuit from non-functioning vent.
    B. Obtain back-up vent and connect vent circuit tubing to it.
    C. Connect $O_2$ line from concentrator to vent.
    D. Check $O_2$ level in blood with pulse oximeter (should be 90% or more).
    E. Unless patient has no functioning vent, 911 will have to be called. Use land line for assistance in emergency tracking – not a cell phone.

## > ____ FIRE:

Reassure patient.  First spreads surprisingly fast.  If you cannot put it out in about 1 minute (using
water, heavy blanket or fire extinguisher that are in rooms or front door), then proceed as follows:

    A.   Call 911 and yell "FIRE" several times to alert others in house.  Scream at the top of your lungs. Disconnect patient from vent and have her breathe through HME only. She can breathe on her own for short periods.

    B.   Drag (using blanket or sheet if possible) or carry her out of the house.

    C.   Let Colette loose outside.

    D.   Do not worry about turning off the $O_2$ supply.


## > ____ CHOKING:

Reassure patient.

    A.   Quickly use in-line catheter to clear inner cannula and trachea.  Use Yankauer catheter to clear
       mouth secretions.

    B.   Position patient to upright Fowler's position.

    C.   If still exhibiting problems, remove inner cannula and replace.

    D.   If inner cannula is clear, but fluid is still entering lungs, inflate trach cuff to 10cc. Patient will not be able to speak, but liquid will stop entering lungs.

    E.   Consider having patient sit up straighter or lie on her side (to drain).

    F.   Call 911 from land line, not cell, to aid in residence location.

# EXHIBIT #4:
# REFERENCE INFORMATION & CONTACTS

## REFERENCE INFORMATION & CONTACTS

**PATIENT INFORMATION:**

Patient Full Name

Full Patient Address, City, State, Zip Code

Patient Home Telephone Number

Patient Date of Birth

Patient Listing of All Allergies:

**MISCELLANEOUS CONTACT INFORMATION:**

Caregiver's Cell Telephone Number .................(807) 555-1111

Caregiver's Work Telephone Number...............(807) 555-2222

Home Care Resources &/or Facilities................(807) 555-3333

**PHYSICIAN & PHARMACY INFORMATION**

Dr. Richard Aaa MD – Neurologist ....................(807) 555-4444

Dr. Loraine Fff, MD – Pulmonologist..................(807) 555-5555

Dr. Frank Ggg, MD – Internist/Primary..............(807) 555-6666

Dr. Mark Ppp, DO – ENT/Otolaryngologist.........(807) 555-7777

Dr. Lucas Sss – Gastroenterologist ....................(807) 555-8888

Pharmacy............................................................(807) 555-9999

**EMERGENCY TRANSPORT INFORMATION:**

Main Dispatch – Available 24/7.......................(807) 555-0000

* If this is <u>NOT</u> an emergency, please request no lights or sirens.
* Advise them that Patient is vent dependent AND that we have: 1) portable vent;  2) portable $O_2$;  3) nurse to accompany them.

**VENT SETTINGS:**

| | |
|---|---|
| Mode:  SIMV | Rate:  10 breaths per minute |
| Tidal Volume:  450 | Pressure Support:  12 |
| Inspiration Time:  1:2 | High Pressure Alarm:  50 |
| Low Pressure Alarm:  3 | PEEP:  3 |
| $O_2$L/Minute Flow: 3L | |

# EXHIBIT #5A:
# MONTHLY NURSING TREATMENT
# FORM PAGE 1

*Monthly Nursing Treatment Form:* Page 1 of 6 (04/2015)

| Patient Name | Erythromycin | | | | | | | | | | | | | | | |
|---|---|---|---|---|---|---|---|---|---|---|---|---|---|---|---|---|
| **Name** | **Allergies** | **For Month / Year** | | | | | **Prepared By** | | | | **Date** | | | | | |
| | | 1 | 2 | 3 | 4 | 5 | 6 | 7 | 8 | 9 | 10 | 11 | 12 | 13 | 14 | 15 | 16 |

**qShift**
Review communication
book at beginning of shift.
Start from your last shift to end of current notations.

**qShift**
1) Check vent circuit &
settings at beginning of shift;
2) obtain vitals; 3) assess trach & peg sites; 4) Document.

**qShift**
Adhere to Universal
Precautions at all times.

**qShift**
Maintain SpO$_2$ ≥95%.
If ≤92%, increase O$_2$ to 4L

**q3-4hours & PRN**
Change undergarments and
inserts. Provide full care including
pulmonary treatment.

| Nurse's Signature | Initials | |
|---|---|---|
| | | |
| | | |

# EXHIBIT #5B:
# MONTHLY NURSING TREATMENT FORM PAGE 3

*Monthly Nursing Treatment Form:* Page 3 of 6 (04/2015)

| Patient Name | Erythromycin | | | | | | | | | | | | | | | |
|---|---|---|---|---|---|---|---|---|---|---|---|---|---|---|---|---|
| **Name** | **Allergies** | **For Month / Year** | | | | | | **Prepared By** | | | | **Date** | | | |
| | | 1 | 2 | 3 | 4 | 5 | 6 | 7 | 8 | 9 | 10 | 11 | 12 | 13 | 14 | 15 | 16 |

| | 1 | 2 | 3 | 4 | 5 | 6 | 7 | 8 | 9 | 10 | 11 | 12 | 13 | 14 | 15 | 16 |
|---|---|---|---|---|---|---|---|---|---|---|---|---|---|---|---|---|
| **qShift @ End** Clean suction machine cannister & tubing at shift end. Insure flush for tubing is available. | | | | | | | | | | | | | | | | |
| **BID & PRN** Perform peg care: Clean w/ $H_2O_2$ **BID**. Apply A&D post cleaning & **PRN**. Cover with split gauze. Insure dressing is dry at all times. | | | | | | | | | | | | | | | | |
| **qDay & PRN** Perform trach care: Cleanse w/1:1 soln NS:$H_2O_2$. Assess skin under ties. Apply medication per MAR Daily Orders. Apply split gauze. | | | | | | | | | | | | | | | | |
| **qDay & PRN** Chg inner cannula & HME. | | | | | | | | | | | | | | | | |
| **q3Day & PRN** Change in-line suction catheter & Flex Connector | | | | | | | | | | | | | | | | |
| **q3Day & PRN** Change trach ties ensuring airway is maintained at all times. | | | | | | | | | | | | | | | | |
| **qWeek & PRN** Wash filters in bedside vent (2 total). | | | | | | | | | | | | | | | | |

| Nurse's Signature | Initials | |
|---|---|---|
| | | |
| | | |

## MONTHLY NURSING TREATMENT FORM PAGE 1
## MONTHLY NURSING TREATMENT FORM PAGE 3

Simply stated, Treatment Forms are a "to-do" list of requirements for the patient's care. Two samples of this patient's six-page document are provided to illustrate various time frames and how to depict when a certain task may require attention.

The **top horizontal line** for Treatment Forms details general information data. This line includes the patient's name, allergies, and the responsible party who completed the form for that particular month. The remaining form documents essential tasks, provides time frames for completion as well as detailing specific actions and care that may be required.

**"Name":** Regardless of whether you have one or multiple patients, this field is crucial as it identifies and highlights the person for whom you are caring. As we had two patients, it is essential. It can also be fundamental for insurance reimbursement.

**"Allergies":** Allergic reactions can be life-threatening and deadly. Allergies to medications and foods are one of the first questions any medical professional will ask. Answers may determine which medications may be administered—but more importantly, which ones may not. And as some medications may be food-based, food allergies are equally important.

**"For Month / Year:"** This field specifies the month and year for which these orders are pertinent. This is a snapshot of what is required for one month—that month only.

**"Prepared By":** The individual completing the Treatment Form initials this field. This is the responsible party who ensures that all that needs to be done is scheduled properly.

**"Date":** Our Treatment and Medication Sheets are typically available during the last week of the prior month. However, changes can occur after the published time. This field provides the date when changes were captured from the previous month. amendments to the forms may be required after that date.

Descriptions and details for the columns appear below. There is some deviation from page one versus page three of the exhibit due to time requirements of the treatments and equipment changes.

**Treatment Specifics:** On both pages 1 and 3 of the exhibits, the first line in first column lists when treatments are to be completed. Timing is depicted by "q(Time)" where "q" refers to the "quantity" of the action or "once per". Therefore, "qShift" would be translated as "once every shift", "qWeek" is translated as "once every week", *etc.* The second and subsequent lines detail what and how to perform the treatments.

**Page 1 of this Exhibit:** Entries illustrate actions which need to be done each and every shift. However, at the end of the page referring to "Undergarment Change", this time is noted as q3-4h, or "once 3 to 4 hours". This specifically states that this task is required every 3 or 4 hours—not merely once per shift.

**Page 3 of this Exhibit:** This illustrates some tasks that must be completed less often than each shift or daily, such as changing Trach Ties, which is completed every 3 days. However, indicating when such action is required is a documentation quandary because completion times vary and not performed each day or every shift. To rectify this, we highlight the day on which the action **IS** required. This is the minimum time frame when this action is necessary. All treatment entries are also classified as "PRN" (meaning when and if necessary) so they may be completed more often if the need arises.

**"1-31":** Although some columns are not present in this exhibit due to space limitations, our form has a numbered column from 1 to 31 to pertain to each day of the month. For all pages, once a treatment is completed, whether per shift, daily, weekly, *etc.*, the caregiver initials the box corresponding to the item under the appropriate date. This signifies that that specific task was completed as required for that specific time.

**"NURSE'S SIGNATURE/INITIALS":** A signature box follows last to identify all nurses who provide care that month. After their signature, they provide initials which are then used to identify the responsible professional who completed, assessed, and documented the action.

# EXHIBIT #6A:
# DAILY MEDICATION ADMINISTRATION RECORD—PAGE 1

*Daily Medication Administration Record:* Page 1 of 8 (08/2015)

| Patient Name | Erythromycin | | | | | | | | | | | | | | | | |
|---|---|---|---|---|---|---|---|---|---|---|---|---|---|---|---|---|---|
| **Name** | **Allergies** | | | **For Month / Year** | | | | | **Prepared By** | | | | **Date** | | | | |
| | Time | 1 | 2 | 3 | 4 | 5 | 6 | 7 | 8 | 9 | 10 | 11 | 12 | 13 | 14 | 15 | 16 |
| **Sucralfate** | 5a | | | | | | | | | | | | | | | | |
| 1gm q6h GT | 11a | | | | | | | | | | | | | | | | |
| | 5p | | | | | | | | | | | | | | | | |
| | 11p | | | | | | | | | | | | | | | | |
| **Ducolax** | 6a | x | x | | x | | x | | x | x | | x | | x | | x | x |
| (Bisacodyl) Supp | | s | sn | m | t | w | th | f | s | sn | m | t | w | th | f | s | sn |

Mon., Wed., Fri per rectum. **NOTE: If no BM in 48 hrs, give Fleet enema per TX order on pg 3.**

| **Replete w/Fiber** | 7a | | | | | | | | | | | | | | | | |
|---|---|---|---|---|---|---|---|---|---|---|---|---|---|---|---|---|---|
| **& Protein** | 12p | | | | | | | | | | | | | | | | |
| | 6p | | | | | | | | | | | | | | | | |
| 12 can @ | 9p | | | | | | | | | | | | | | | | |
| 12 can @ | 11p | | | | | | | | | | | | | | | | |

Admin as slow bolus. Total of 4-250 mL feedings daily GT. **MIX with 100mL** H₂0 R/T thickness

| **Norvasc** | 9a | | | | | | | | | | | | | | | | |
|---|---|---|---|---|---|---|---|---|---|---|---|---|---|---|---|---|---|
| 2.5mg BID GT | 11p | | | | | | | | | | | | | | | | |

*Hold if systolic<90.*

| **Systolic BP** | 9a | | | | | | | | | | | | | | | | |
|---|---|---|---|---|---|---|---|---|---|---|---|---|---|---|---|---|---|
| pre-administration | 11p | | | | | | | | | | | | | | | | |

*of Norvasc*

| Nurse's Signature | Initials | |
|---|---|---|
| | | |
| | | |
| | | |

# EXHIBIT #6B:
# PRN MEDICATION ADMINISTRATION
# RECORD—PAGE 6

*PRN Medication Administration Record:* Page 6 of 8 (08/2015)

| Patient Name | Erythromycin | | | | | | | | | | | | | | | | | |
|---|---|---|---|---|---|---|---|---|---|---|---|---|---|---|---|---|---|---|
| **Name** | **Allergies** | | For Month / Year | | | | | | | Prepared By | | | | Date | | | | |
| | | **1** | **2** | **3** | **4** | **5** | **6** | **7** | **8** | **9** | **10** | **11** | **12** | **13** | **14** | **15** | **16** | |
| **Lidoderm 5%** | On | | | | | | | | | | | | | | | | | |
| **Transderm Patch** | Initials | | | | | | | | | | | | | | | | | |
| 0.5-1 patcH QD PRN | Off | | | | | | | | | | | | | | | | | |
| topically for pain. | Initials | | | | | | | | | | | | | | | | | |
| Apply max 12hr on - | L or R | | | | | | | | | | | | | | | | | |
| 12 hrs off prior to | Site | | | | | | | | | | | | | | | | | |
| next application. | | | | | | | | | | | | | | | | | | |
| **Ativan** | Time | | | | | | | | | | | | | | | | | |
| 0.5mg x1 PRN GT for | Initials | | | | | | | | | | | | | | | | | |
| anxiety. | | | | | | | | | | | | | | | | | | |
| **Nasocort** | Time | | | | | | | | | | | | | | | | | |
| i-ii sprays QD PRN | Amt | | | | | | | | | | | | | | | | | |
| nasal for allergies. | Initials | | | | | | | | | | | | | | | | | |
| **Benadryl** | Time | | | | | | | | | | | | | | | | | |
| 12.5mg QD PRN | Initials | | | | | | | | | | | | | | | | | |
| GT for allergies. | | | | | | | | | | | | | | | | | | |
| **Fleet Liq Gylcerin** | Time | | | | | | | | | | | | | | | | | |
| Supp 7.5mL PRN | Initials | | | | | | | | | | | | | | | | | |
| rectal for constipation. | | | | | | | | | | | | | | | | | | |

| Nurse's Signature | Initials | |
|---|---|---|
| | | |
| | | |

Often referred to as the "MAR", the Medication Administration Record follows the same pattern as the treatment form. However, instead of the activities which need to be performed in column 1, the administration of medications and feedings are noted.

Again, only a sample of the MAR is provided: the first and sixth pages of eight, in this patient's case, are shown.

The **top horizontal** line of the MAR is exactly the same as that for the Treatment Sheets and details just general patient and completion information. This line includes the patient's name, allergies, and the responsible party who completed the form for that particular month.

**"Name":** Regardless of whether you have one or multiple patients, this field is crucial as it identifies and highlights the person for whom you are caring. As we had two patients, it is essential. It can also be fundamental for insurance reimbursement.

**"Allergies":** Allergic reactions can be life-threatening and deadly. Allergies to medications and foods are one of the first questions any medical professional will ask. Answers may determine which medications may be administered—but more importantly, which ones may not. And as some medications may be food-based, food allergies are equally important.

**"For Month / Year:"** This field specifies the month and year for which these orders are pertinent. This is a snapshot of what is required for one month—that month only.

**"Prepared By":** The individual completing the Medication Form initials this field. This is the responsible party who ensures that all medications are scheduled properly.

**"Date":** Our Treatment and Medication Sheets are typically available during the last week of the prior month. However, changes can occur after the published time. This field provides the date when changes were captured from the previuos month.

Column descriptions follow next:

**MEDICATION SPECIFICS:** On Page One of the exhibit, the first column lists the medication in bold typeface (**Sucralfate,** e.g.). Below the medication, the dosage amount to be administered each time is provided (1gram) as well as how often through-out the day (q6h=every 6 hours), and the route (GT=via gastric tube). Notes and directions for a medication's administration may also be provided, as is noted for the medication "Norvasc." The physician has ordered that this medication should not be given if a blood pressure reading is too low ("hold if systolic is less than 90").

Page Six of the MAR is the same as Page One, including medication name, amount, timing, and notes if applicable. However, in addition to this information, a PRN medication, which is only given as needed, also includes "why" it is given, such as for pain, allergies, rash.

**"TIME":** Page One is straightforward. It lists the time of day that the medication is given to the patient based upon the physician orders. "Sucralfate" is to be given every 6 hours at 5a.m., 11a.m., 5p.m. and 10:30p.m., plus or minus one hour.

Page Six does not list times because these medications are to be administered only when needed and at no specific time. Under this column there appear two standard fields: **TIME and IN-TIALS.** If the patient was feeling congested for example, Benadryl could be given. The nurse or caregiver would simply complete the time it was given and provide her initials.

However, in addition to time and initials, some medications require qualifiers which may include dosages or locations. For example, one or two sprays of "Nasacort" may be given for allergy relief. The amount that was instilled, the number of sprays, would then be noted under "**AMT.**" Topical medications require information as to what part of the body they were applied. "Lidoderm Patch" is used for pain, and it must be stated under "**SITE**" where the patch was applied, such as "arm" or "back" for example, and a designation of "left" or "right" under "**L/R**", when pertinent. In addition, this specific medication requires removal after 12 hours. Therefore, the time it was applied and the time it was removed must both be recorded.

"**1-31**": Although some columns are not present in this exhibit due to space limitations, our form has a numbered column from 1 to 31 to pertain to each day of the month. For all pages, once a treatment is completed, whether per shift, daily, weekly, *etc.*, the caregiver initials the box corresponding to the item under the appropriate date. This signifies that that specific task was completed as required for that specific time.

**"NURSE'S SIGNATURE/INITIALS"**: A signature box follows last to identify all nurses who provide care that month. After their signature, they provide initials which are then used to identify the responsible professional who completed, assessed, and documented the action.

# EXHIBIT #7A:
# NURSING REVIEW / ASSESSMENT
# FORM PAGE 1

## NURSING REVIEW / ASSESSMENT FORM FOR "PATIENT" - PAGE 1 OF 2 (08/2015)

**DATE:** __ / __ / __    **DAY:** SU M T W TH F SA    **SHIFT:** ____ TO ____    **LPN/RN:** _____

**V/S** TIME: _____ BP: _____ / _____ HR: _____ RR: _____ O₂ SAT: _____ TEMP: _____ PAIN: _____

_____ _____ / _____ _____ _____ _____ _____ _____

_____ _____ / _____ _____ _____ _____ _____ _____

**VENT SETTINGS:** Mode: _____    Rate: _____    Tidal Volume: _____

Pressure Support: _____    Inspiration Time: _____    High Pressure Alarm: _____

Low Pressure Alarm: _____    PEEP: _____    O₂ Line Secure: Y / N

O₂ Liter Flow: _____    O₂ Water Level: _____    Cuff Inflation: _____cc

**INTAKE:** TIME:    FEEDING:    YOGURT:    CRANBERRY:    FREE H₂O:    DILUTED MEDS IN H₂O:

_____ _____ _____ _____ _____ _____

_____ _____ _____ _____ _____ _____

_____ _____ _____ _____ _____ _____

_____ _____ _____ _____ _____ _____

TOTALS: _____ _____ _____ _____ _____    **SHIFT TOTAL:** _____

**NEUROLOGY:** 1) MENTAL STATUS: A A OX__ Lethargic @ ___ / Sleepy @ ___ / Appropriate @___ / Anxious @ ___ /
Repetitive @ ____ / Confused @____ / Forgetful @ ____ / Other _____ @_____ MEDS GIVEN? Y / N
2) SPEECH: Clear @ ____ / Slurred – Mumbled @ _____ / Difficult @ _____ / Unable @ _____ / Wet @ _____ /
Other _____ @ _____ 3) CHANGES DURING SHIFT: _____
4) ADDL INFO: _____

**RESPIRATORY:** 1) LUNG SOUNDS - Time: _____ Description: _____
_____ _____
2) SUCTION - Time: _____ x ____ VIA Trach / Oral / Nasal Quantity: _____ Quality: _____
_____ x ____ VIA Trach / Oral / Nasal _____ _____
_____ x ____ VIA Trach / Oral / Nasal _____ _____
3) EQUIP CHGD A) HME: Y / N B) Inner Cannula: Y / N C) Ties: Y / N D) Dsg: Y / N E) In-Line-Cath: Y / N
4) TRACH - Stoma Site: _____ Skin Under Ties: _____
Care / TX: _____
5) ADDL INFO _____

**CARDIOVASCULAR:** 1) HR REGULAR: Y / N 2) EDEMA: Y / N : Location: _____ 3) CAP REFILL ≤ 3 SEC: Y / N
4) PEDAL PULSES: Regular Equal / Weak / Absent / Unilateral SPECIFY _____ 5) RADIAL PULSES: _____
6) ADDL INFO: _____

**Assessments are crucial for evaluating and appraising a patient.** It provides a history of the patient's medical condition, which then allows for comparisons as well as to understand what is normal for that person. **Ten individual system categories for this patient are assessed and/or documented by the utilization of this assessment form** and at the **beginning of each nursing shift**, the oncoming nurse begins completion of a new document.

- **SHIFT DETAILS:** This area merely defines the specifics of one particular nursing shift. This includes the **date, day** and **shift details**. In addition, a line is available for the nurse to **PRINT** their last name for legibility. This line is not intended to be a signature line as that appears at the conclusion of this document.
- **"V/S":** Vital signs (V/S) are numeric measurements that provide a quick evaluation of the patient. By comparing the patient's values to those established as typical of normal healty individuals and populations, insight to the patient's status is provided. Changes in these values over time provide clues to acute changes which may require immediate attention or longer-term consideration for changes in treatments or medications.

  **Additionally, when evaluating the measurements together, they can alert nurses to possible problem situations,** such as shock, when blood pressure is low combined with a rapid heart rate. However, changes in signs could also be due to improperly placed equipment. If one of the values is abnormal for the patient, it should be taken again to determine if it is repeatable or merely an erroneous reading. In addition, although typical values for an adult are representative for the majority of the population, each individual differs. Therefore, what may be abnormal for the general population may be perfectly normal for a different individual.

**Equipment is required to obtain some vital signs such as blood pressure and the oxygen saturation of the blood.** To obtain a **heart rate,** a watch and palpation of the artery can be used. The **respiration rate,** similarly, can be obtained with a watch and observing the number of breaths. An increase in **temperature** can be determined by the touch of a hand to a forehead. The following are noted and obtained as follows:

> **"TIME":** The **time of day** that the vital signs are taken is indicated.

> **"B/P":** This records **blood pressure,** which may be obtained by an automatic wrist cuff unit or via a stethoscope and sphygmomanometer. Blood pressure is used in evaluating cardiac output and fluid volume, for example. Unusually high or low readings or great variability can be causes for concern.

**Two values are noted in blood pressure readings: for example, 120mmHg/70mmHg.** The values are pressure units in terms of the pressure exerted by a column of mercury (Hg) at an indicated height. **The first number (120mmHg) is the systolic blood pressure** and represents **the pressure that the blood flow exerts on the walls of**

the arteries when the heart contracts, or pumps. **A normal value in most adult patients is considered to be in a range from 100-140mmHg,** but values over 120mmHg may be monitored, as they might be considered a pre-hypertension value, warning of potentially chronic high blood pressure. The second number (70mmHg) reflects **the pressure that is exerted on those vessels when the heart is not pumping but resting, the diastolic blood pressure. For adults, this value is typically 50-80mmHg.**

> **"HR":** The **heart rate, the number of times the heart beats in one minute,** can be obtained in multiple ways. Often it is measured when using other instrumentation, such as a wrist blood pressure cuff or pulse oximeter. It can also be obtained using a watch with a second hand and feeling a pulse. Numerous pulse points could be used but the radial pulse at the wrist is regularly and most easily felt and recognized. **The value for a normal adult is usually between 60 and 100 beats per minute.**

> **"RR":** The **respiration rate is simply the number of breaths that are taken in one minute** and requires no equipment to measure except a watch with a second hand to count the number of times the patient breathes. If the respirations, or breaths, are shallow, placing a hand on the patient's chest can aid in obtaining the value. A recognized normal value for respirations is 16 to 20 breaths each minute, for a resting patient.

> **"$O_2$ Sat":** Abbreviated for **oxygen saturation (or $SaO_2$), this is the percentage of the red blood cells that are rich in oxygen located in the arteries.** This reflects

the effectiveness of respiration and oxygen transfer from the lungs to the blood. This vital sign requires use of a **pulse oximeter** to obtain the measurement and often the heart rate is a secondary measure that is also provided. **A value at or above 96% without supplemental oxygen is considered normal.**

> **"Temp": The body temperature provides an indicator of disease processes versus health.** Unusually high values (fever) indicate infection of some type. There are numerous ways to obtain body temperature readings such as **orally, tympanic (by ear), rectal or axillary (armpit). For each method, normal values differ.** For example a rectal reading may be one degree higher than those obtained orally, and axillary measurements not only take a long time to obtain, but may also be lower by one degree. Whatever location is used, this should be the only method used, for patient accuracy and comparison purposes. In addition, it should be noted that normal body temperatures not only vary by body location, but also can vary up to two degrees depending on the time of day.

> **"Pain": Using a pain scale assists in providing a qualitative measure of the patient's discomfort.** Often used as a rating from 0 to 10, where 0 is no pain and 10 is the worst possible pain, the patient provides his pain number. By having such a guide, it can be determined not only if, but when and what pain medication or treatments should be offered.

- **"VENT SETTINGS": Used for ventilator-dependent**

patients with pulmonary problems, vent settings are dictated by a pulmonologist.

> **"Mode":** How the ventilator works is indicated under this field, ventilator mode. **There are numerous types of modes ranging from those that initiate all breaths to those that provide breaths only if necessary.** Some of these modes include Control Ventilation, Assist-Control Ventilation, Continuous Mandatory Ventilation, and Synchronous Intermittent Mandatory Ventilation. Depending on the mode used, other criteria may or may not be preset or utilized.

> **"Rate": This is the preset minimum number of breaths that the machine will deliver to the patient per minute.** Breaths may be delivered if the patient doesn't take as many as is dictated by the rate. Then the machine will provide the extra. In some cases, the machine solely provides respiration when patients are unable to breathe for themselves.

> **"Tidal Volume":** This is the volume of oxygen that the patient receives or exhales. Depending on the machine, this could either be the amount of gas that is delivered or the amount of exhaled volume measured at a particular point on the ventilator tubing.

> **"Pressure Support": Pressure support ventilation is used to assist a patient's own self-driven breathing effort.** By reducing the work of breathing, the patient is made more comfortable and able to take more spontaneous breaths. While still maintaining preset limits for

volume and rate, and including positive pressure, the patient controls machine activity by actively breathing.

> **"Inspiration Time":** This actually is a **ratio of the inspiration time versus expiration duration.** With settings usually at a 1:1.5 or 1:2 ratio, the duration of the inspiration is typically less than the amount of time used for exhalation, as is typically normal during a non-ventilated breathing cycle.

> **"High Pressure Alarm":** This is the pressure at which an alarm for high pressure measured by the vent will sound. High pressure could be the result of a kink in the tubing. In some instances, increases in pressure above the limit are caused by the presence of a mucus plug or merely by coughing or yawning.

> **"Low Pressure Alarm": A low pressure alarm will sound when pressures are not sufficient and is typically a more life-threatening situation than a high-pressure condition.** While the vent is in operation, sensors identify constant positive and negative pressures, similar to what the diaphragm does naturally. **Low pressure alarms typically sound when the patient has become disconnected from the vent.**

> **"Peep":** Abbreviation for "positive end-expiratory pressure," this is the **positive pressure left in the alveoli of the lungs at the end of expiration, or exhaled breaths.** The pressure improves oxygenation by ensuring these very small functional units of the lungs are not fully collapsed, making it easier to expand during the next inspiration.

> **"O₂ Line Secure":** By circling "Y" for "Yes" or "N" for "No," the nurse indicates that the oxygen line connecting the vent to the oxygen supply, typically a concentrator, has been checked and is securely attached.

> **"O₂ Liter Flow":** This is the volume of oxygen (in liters) delivered to the patient per minute via an outside source. A liter is 1.1 quarts.

> **"O₂ Water Level":** This abbreviated field pertains to the oxygen source, a concentrator, which **has a bubbler to humidify the oxygen before it flows to the patient.** Air that is not humidified is dry and can potentially be irritating, causing pulmonary tissue sensitivity. By having a humidification source that adds moisture to the oxygen released from the concentrator, dryness problems are greatly eliminated. This field is to ensure the water is checked each shift and maintained at the proper level specifically indicated on the bubbler bottles.

> **"Cuff Inflation __ cc":** This patient has a tracheostomy, a small tube inserted through the front of the neck and into the windpipe (trachea). To hold the trach tube in place, air is instilled into a balloon within the unit. If air is not present, the balloon is completely deflated, and the trach would not stay in place. The amount of air instilled is dependent on many factors, including enabling vocalization and activity. The balloon is checked each shift to ensure safety, and the amount of air that was instilled is indicated in this field.

- **"INTAKE": The amount the patient ingests is vital to**

**know.** This is true whether the patient has a gastric tube or ingests all nutrition and fluids by mouth.

**The intake section of this form is for a patient who receives all nutrition and fluids via a gastric tube** primarily to prevent aspiration pneumonia caused by food, fluids, or vomitus entering the trachea and thus entering the pulmonary system instead of going into the esophagus and gastrointestinal system. This patient is considered "NPO", Latin *nil per os*, translated as "nothing by mouth".

The fields in this section of the Assessment Form are generally self-explanatory. They include the **time** the substance was given as well as a breakdown of **what** was given with the volume in milliliters (mL).

This patient receives **feedings** via a gastric-tube which is a complete liquid nutrition that provides protein, fiber, minerals and other essential ingredients to sustain life. In addition, also via the gastric-tube, she is administered **yogurt** (kefir), **cranberry juice**, and water. **Free water** is the amount of water that is provided by the nurse over and above what is required on the medication administration record ("MAR").

**Totals** for each category are completed at the end of the shift. A summed **shift total** for all categories added together completes this section.

- **"NEUROLOGIC":** In general, two main criteria are assessed for this patient. These include mental status and speech. However, it should be noted that additional neurological functions can be assessed depending on the patient. The functions on which we concentrate are highlighted below.

> **"1) Mental Status"**: Various terms are provided to describe the mental status of this patient. In addition to a specific term, a section is provided to indicate the time at which this condition was noted (@_____). At the end of the field "Meds given Y/N" is provided to ensure an efficient method of capturing whether medication was given to decrease any adverse situation and/or to calm the patient, as would be the case with administration of Ativan, for example. This field only pertains to anti-anxiety medications the patient may have on order.

> **"2) Speech"**: At times, this patient has difficulty in vocalization. An assessment of speech is done throughout each shift. Again, the time which such a condition is noted after the "@" sign.

> **"3) Changes during Shift"**: During a short period of time, neurological changes can present often and frequently. For example, a patient may be sleepy in the morning and confused. As the day progresses, he might become forgetful. In the evening, to orient himself, he might exhibit an involuntary repetition of words or phrases that were heard (echolalia), and may become anxious with this action. This field, used in conjunction with "1) Mental Status" provides additional space to note such variances in abilities or moods and is dedicated solely to that purpose.

> **"4) Addl Info":** Space is available at the end of the section to highlight additional information that may be pertinent and specific to this system only, the patient's neurology functioning, for ease in capturing and reviewing.

For this patient, who is quadriplegic with sensory and motor function impairments, there is limited neurology assessment, and it involves mental status and speech only. However, for other patients many other criteria could be assessed. These include the following.

**Cranial Nerves** function in sensory and motor abilities, such as eye movement, chewing, swallowing, taste, facial expressions, and gag and corneal reflexes; **Sensory Function** assess ability to sense or perceive in various areas sensations such as pain, light touch, vibration, position, and discriminate objects or touch on the patient's body; **Motor Function** tests muscle tone and range of motion, muscle strength by observation of gait and muscle resistance tests, as well as coordination; and **Reflexes,** such as deep tendon reflexes at the bicep, patella (knee), and Achilles tendon and superficial reflexes that respond when tickling the feet and abdomen.

- **RESPIRATORY: This section is used to assess and detail pulmonary function and changes throughout the shift.**

> **"1) Lung Sounds":** Often referred to as "breath sounds," this provides for sounds heard when listening to the lung fields (asculation) with a stethoscope. While clear sounds are ideal, abnormal breath sounds are often

heard. The time assessed and the descriptions of the sounds are noted.

**The most common abnormal breath sounds include:** 1) **Rhonchi:** heard in the larger airways usually during expiration but at times during inspiration; often disappear when the patient coughs or is suctioned; are low-pitched, rattling, and similar to snoring; 2) **Wheezes**: heard during expiration usually but when more severe also during inspiration; often musical and high-pitched; do not disappear during suctioning or coughing; 3) **Crackles:** heard during inspiration usually; result from alveoli popping open; classified as either fine (occur in the lung bases when inhaling stops and sound similar to hair being rubbed between fingers) or coarse (occur throughout lungs when inhaling starts and sound similar to bubbling or gurgling).

> **"2) Suction":** This ventilator-dependent patient requires suctioning to clear larger airways of secretions. The time is noted when suction is provided as well as the number of times it was necessary to eliminate mucus that could block the airways.

**Suctioning may be accomplished in three ways and the method used is circled. The in-line suction catheter** provides a sterile self-contained unit which enters the trach opening (stoma) directly to the bronchus of the lungs. The catheter is attached to a suction unit and advanced to remove fluid and mucus. **Oral suction** is accomplished by using an oral suction device, often a Yankauer tube unit that is also attached to a suction machine and placed in the oral cavity. The **nasal** method is used with the suction machine tubing only, placed close to the nostrils (nares).

**The quantity of the suctioned secretions is indicated.** Descriptive terms such as "scant," "moderate," and "large" are often used because the actual amount cannot be measured.

**The quality of the secretions is perhaps the more meaningful of the descriptions, as it provides a bigger picture of the patient's pulmonary status.** Secretions from the chest are thicker in nature than oral secretions. Color can vary from clear to white to tan to yellow to green. Such differences can lend understanding about infectious processes or indicate they are merely oral secretions (saliva) that have migrated from the mouth. Secretions from the mouth are usually thin and clear, while those of the nasal cavity can also provide infection information.

> **"3) EQUIP CHGD":** To ensure proper care and functioning of the trach, vent, and tracheostomy stoma site, equipment changes are required. Although equipment change intervals are dictated by the Treatment Sheets, **this is also included to provide reminders of required actions and ease in referencing if they were done.** The nurse indicates if the equipment was changed by circling "Y" for "yes" if it was changed or "N" for "not replaced." Depending on the clinical situation, such as during allergy seasons for example, these particular items could be frequently changed if mucus is clogging the inner cannula or secretions are causing the dressing to become frequently wet.

**> "3A) HME": This is an abbreviation for "Heat, Moisture Exchanger."** It is a small piece of ventilator tubing with a deep bed filter that is attached between its sections. The purpose of this is to deliver filtered, moist, warmed air to the patient. The filter also ensures that any secretions from the trach stoma do not advance into the ventilator tubing during exhalation

**> "3B) Inner Cannula": This patient had a procedure, a tracheostomy, performed to provide an airway.** This surgical opening of the trachea provides a hole which then holds equipment to provide entry for mechanical ventilation. This is necessary when pulmonary function and muscles could no longer perform respiration, the act of breathing in and out.

**An opening through the throat and the trachea is surgically made, and an outer tube is inserted into that hole (stoma).** The outer tube has a flange to ensure it remains in place against the skin to prevent it from completely entering the stoma. A balloon cuff surrounds a section of the outer tube placed into the trachea and is filled with a designated amount of air. Therefore, the combination of the flange and balloon cuff holds the unit in place. The trach tube is further secured in position by trach ties which are attached to each end of the flange and circle behind the neck.

**Although this outer tube is changed by a physician at regular intervals, a smaller tube is placed inside this tube.** This smaller tube is called an "inner cannula," and it is replaced daily at a minimum, using sterile technique. **The inner cannula's purpose is to ensure the airway does not become blocked, by providing a barrier between the outer tube and tracheal secretions.** Often it may require more frequent changes, as it can become lined with mucus or clogged, which minimizes or prevents oxygen from entering the trachea and lungs. Each shift indicates what occurred with this during their shift.

> **"3C) Ties":** Trach **ties are also used to hold the outer trach tube in place, in addition to the flange and the balloon cuff.** The trach tie, one long piece of fabric, is placed behind the neck. Each end is then attached to openings at each side of the flange on the outer tube to secure its position. The extra length unnecessary to maintain a fixed position is then folded over and secured by Velcro onto itself, or some other securing mechanism. **Care must be taken to ensure the ties are not secured too tightly or too loosely, allowing for movement, and generally judged by the ease in inserting a finger between the ties and skin.**

> **"3D) Dsg":** To trap secretions and provide cushioning, **a dressing is placed between the skin of the throat and the flange of the outer trach tube.** Split gauze dressings are the preferred dressings to use because they are pre-cut for ease in placement. In addition, the pre-cut edges are sealed intact to prevent bits of fiber from entering the trachea. When removed, the old dressing is evaluated for discharge (exudates), blood, and secretions, and these are documented

> **"3E) In-Line-Cath":** To ease suctioning patients while

**ensuring sterile technique, a closed in-line suction catheter is used.** Attached to the inner cannula at the stoma opening, a thin suction tubing enters the trachea when advanced inward. When at the proper level, suction is applied to remove any secretions that may lie anywhere within the airway.

> **"4) TRACH":** Daily assessment is required to ensure skin integrity of the trach stoma, around the flange, and under the trach ties. Skin under the ties may become inflamed if the ties are too tight, or a rash may develop from moisture that may migrate from secretions or sweat. The stoma and area under the flange could also become boggy with secretions, reddened or bruised (ecchymotic), or generally irritated by the movement of gauze moving against the skin. In addition, the area should be evaluated for discharge or signs of inflammation or infection.

> **"Trach—Stoma Site": The area directly under the flange and surrounding the stoma should be evaluated each shift.** Descriptive terms should indicate color of the skin, any abnormalities, if discharge was present, odor, and general appearance.

> **"Skin Under Ties": The skin under the ties should be assessed each shift.** While providing information concerning the condition of the area, it also ensures that the tautness of the ties is proper. If they are too tight, breakdown could occur, and if too loose, this decreases the functionality of the trach.

> **"Care / TX": Treatment orders from the physician**

**provide for daily care of the site.** Typically, care involves cleaning the site as the physician directs, and applying a split gauze dressing inserted between the neck skin and the flange. Medicated ointments may also be ordered by the physician for application in and around the stomal area. If care is a daily treatment only and was already provided, later shifts may indicate a dressing change if it was wet and required changing or that the dressing was clean, dry, and intact, abbreviated as "CDI."

> **"5) Addl Info": Space is available at the end of the section to highlight additional information** that may be pertinent and specific to this system only, the patient's pulmonary functioning, for ease in capturing and reviewing.

- **CARDIOVASCULAR: This section is used to assess and detail cardiac and venous function and changes throughout the shift.**

> **"1) HR Regular": A regular heart rate simply means that the beating of the heart occurs in a regular rhythm** just as a music has a regular pace and tempo. The number of beats isn't the focal point and isn't counted here, but rather the assessment is whether the heart pumps at a standard cadence and expected time. This information can be obtained by feeling the pulse with fingertips or listening to heart sounds with a stethoscope. Whichever method is used, the rhythm regularity is determined by touch or hearing for 15 seconds. If it is perceived as not being regular, the process is continued for one minute to ensure it is indeed irregular and to determine if there is

any pattern to the irregularity. If the rate is regular, "Y" (yes) is circled.

> **"2) Edema": Edema is a condition where excess fluid is trapped between the tissues.** It is caused numerous ways including gravity, decreased functioning of venous valves, fluid imbalance causing or due to sodium retention, kidney malfunction, cardiac dysfunction, and many other processes. During each shift, edema is assessed by placing a fingertip against skin over a bony prominence. It is pushed down for 5 seconds, then released. If the tissue does not return to normal appearance immediately, edema is present and indicated by circling "Y" (yes). Locations and any qualifying descriptions or grading are provided.

> **"3) Cap Refill <3 Sec": Capillary refill in the fingernails and toenails is another cardiac determinant which is assessed.** Pressure is exerted on the nails then released. The nail bed should go from white to its normal color in three seconds or less. This is a gauge of oxygen perfusion and should be performed not only on the nails on the fingers but also the toes, which are farthest from the heart. When there is inadequate perfusion, oxygenated blood doesn't reach all the tissue. Lack of perfusion for extended periods of time results in tissue death. If the nail beds return to normal color in less than or equal to three seconds, "Y" (yes) is circled.

> **"4) Pedal Pulses": Pedal pulses are simply those pulses that are felt at the feet, which are the most distant pulses from the heart.** Pulses can provide distinct insights

about a beating heart by assessing the rate, rhythm and amplitude of a pulse, which is the blood ejected from the heart during each contraction. While feeling a pulse, the number of beats can be counted, giving heart rate information, although this not documented in this section. Descriptions such as "regular" or "irregular" are used to refer to the regularity of each beat—is the rhythm the same each time or is there a variance among beats? Additionally, pulses offer a qualitative measure concerning the strength or amplitude of blood within the arteries. This can yield information concerning blood deficit (hypovolemia) or conversely blood overload (hypervolemia) as well as cardiac and venous abnormalities and infection processes. These may be described in words and or numbers such as "absent" (0), "weak" or "thready" (+1), "normal" (+2), or "bounding" (+3).

Both the left and right foot pulses should be assessed to determine functioning on both sides of the body. Once palpated, one or more descriptive terms are circled: 1) **Regular** refers to a regular rhythm and rate; 2) **Equal** indicates that the pulses are equal between each foot; are bilaterally present, and the same; 3) **Weak** may be applied to both pulses compared to other pulses in the body, or one side may be weaker than the other; 4) **Absent:** is defined as not (felt) palpable, and if considered absent, both pedal pulses on the same foot should be assessed; 5) **Unilateral** means "one sided only" and is used when there is a difference between the feet, that is the conditions appears on the right only or the left only. Space is available for any notation.

> **"5) Radial Pulses":** To provide comparison with the pedal pulses, radial pulses are assessed. **The radial pulses are felt around the wrist level at the back of the arm, the palm side, originating from the thumb.** Again, both radial pulses should be checked to determine if pulsations are equal. The results are documented using descriptions as noted under "Pedal Pulses".

> **"6) Addl Info":** Space is available at the end of the section to highlight additional information** that may be pertinent and specific to this system only, the patient's cardiovascular functioning, for ease in capturing and reviewing.

# EXHIBIT #7B:
# NURSING REVIEW / ASSESSMENT
# FORM PAGE 2

**NURSING REVIEW / ASSESSMENT FORM FOR "PATIENT" - PAGE 2 OF 2** (08/2015)

**GASTROINTESTINAL:** 1) BOWEL SOUNDS: Present x ___ / Sluggish / Quiet / Hyperactive / Hypoactive / Absent /
Qualify if not 4 quad: ____ 2) ABDOMEN: Soft / Firm / Tender / Non-Tender / Distended / Firm / Other: _____
3) PEG: A) Tube Patent: Y / N  B) Feeding Held: Y / N  4) PEG SITE: A) Dsg CDI: Y / N (Desc if No) _____
B) Site:_____
C) Care/TX: _____
5) STOOL: A) BM During Shift: Y / N  B) Notes: _____
6) OTHER: A) Nausea: Y / N  B) Emesis: Y / N  C) Other: _____
7) ADDL INFO: _____

**GENITOURINARY:** Time: _____ Saturation: _____ Odor: _____ Full Chg: Y / N Insert: Removed / Placed
_____ _____ _____ Y / N Removed / Placed
_____ _____ _____ Y / N Removed / Placed
_____ _____ _____ Y / N Removed / Placed
*) ADDL INFO: _____

**MUSCULOSKELETAL / SKIN:** 1) DESCRIPTION: warm / hot / cool / cold / dry / moist / diaphoretic / color: _____
2) CONDITION: A) Intact: Y / N  B) Dsg Locations & Types: _____
C) Wound Descr: _____
D) TX: _____
3) CARE: pericare / bath / hair washed / A&D (area) _____ Lotion (area) _____
4) T&P on right side at (time): _____ _____ _____ _____ _____
5) OOB VIA HOYER TO WC: Y / N - duration: _____ 6) PRURITUS: Y / N - area & TX: _____ 7) PROM: Y / N
8) ADDL INFO: _____

**PSYCHO/SOCIAL:** 1) PT CONCERNS: _____ 2) SLEEP / REST: _____
3) MOOD / DISPOSITION: A) Beginning Shift: _____ B) End Shift:_____
4) ADDL INFO: _____
_____

**NOTES:** _____
_____
_____
_____
_____
_____
_____

**NURSE'S SIGNATURE:** _____

- **GASTROINTESTINAL: This section is used to assess and detail the gastrointestinal, often abbreviated as "GI" system, function and changes throughout the shift.**

  **Patients who do not obtain nutrition by mouth require all substances for survival be directly received into the stomach or the jejunum section of the small intestine via a tube placed surgically. This patient had a percutaneous endoscopic gastrostomy (PEG) which is a tube placed into the stomach to deliver fluids and nutrition. From the stomach, it extends out through the stomach wall, muscles, and skin, to the outside of the body.** Daily care and assessment is essential for the continued functioning of the tube, and this section is used to assess and detail gastrointestinal changes throughout the shift.

  > **"1) Bowel Sounds":** The noise that occurs when your stomach growls, especially before meals, are bowel sounds. When air or food contents move through the large intestine (the colon) by contraction of the muscular wall (peristalsis), sounds can be heard. **Each shift assesses for bowel sounds with a stethoscope.**

  The colon is generally shaped like an upside-down U and four sections of this "U" (the two ends and corners of the "U") are assessed. These are known as "quadrants." Beginning to the right and below the belly-button (umbilicus), the progression is then to move above right of the umbilicus, to above left and finally below left of the umbilicus. Sounds often are detected soon. But if they appear absent, extra time should be spent in that area.

Documentation includes the following information referring to activity of the sounds and their presence. More than one adjective may be circled and used together for full description.

**"Present x___":** indicate if sounds are present in 1, 2, 3 or all 4 quadrants. If no other selection is circled, then the sounds are considered normal.

**"Sluggish":** refers to long, slow sounds that are intermittently present.

**"Quiet":** describes sounds that are present but not loud.

**"Hyperactive":** occur rapidly; are loud, high-pitched sounds often associated with hunger; also present with diarrhea or laxative use.

**"Hypoactive":** are not heard frequently and require time to be fully ascultated; often associated with sluggish or quiet bowel sounds; can indicate a bowel obstruction or decreased peristalsis, which could lead to constipation or diverticulitis.

**"Absent":** when the quadrant is listened to for several minutes and no sound is heard; this can indicate bowel obstruction or torsion of the bowel, known as "paralytic ileus," potentially life-threatening.

**"Qualify as needed if not 4Quads":** since bowel sounds can vary from quadrant to quadrant, indicate where any abnormal bowel sounds are noted.

**> "2) Abdomen": The abdomen is observed and lightly palpated.** This should be done after bowel sounds are ascultated (heard via stethoscope) as palpation could affect the natural quality of the sounds. A typical normal assessment is **soft** and **non-tender.** Abnormal findings are "**firm**" and "**distended**," which may indicate excess stool, constipation, or bleeding. If the area is tender or painful, along with distention or firmness, further assessment is required. It should be noted that distention and firmness could also be positional—depending on the patient's position in bed. By changing the position, these characteristics could change. If gas is suspected and the patient has a PEG tube, by opening the top, trapped air may be released. The pertinent descriptive term is circled.

**> "3) PEG":** This patient has a gastric tube in place for delivery of nutrition and fluids. This section pertains to this particular situation.

**> "3A) Tube Patent":** If fluid runs freely through the tube, it is considered patent and "Y" is indicated. If the tube is not patent, and therefore not functioning and unusable, then "N" is circled.

**> "3B) Feeding Held":** Feedings are deliberately not administered for various reasons. They include excess residual left from the previous feeding, which indicates digestion is delayed. This must be monitored. Delay may also be due to a physician's wanting to ensure there are no gastric contents if the tube is going to be changed or for some other procedure on the body when anesthesia may be administered. If one feeding was held, even if additional nutrients were given during the shift, "Y" for "yes" should be circled. Clarifying explanations should be provided under "Addl Info".

> **"4) PEG Site:** The location where the tube exits the body is called the "PEG site". This hole extends from the top layer of skin, through fat and muscles, and ultimately concludes in the stomach area. The area requires assessment each shift, as stomach contents, inflammatory discharge, bleeding, or other fluids could escape from this stoma.

> **"4A) Dressing—CDI":** At the beginning of the shift, an indication is made whether the dressing to the PEG site was clean, dry, and intact (abbreviated by "CDI"). If it was, then "Y" for 'yes' is indicated. If it is not CDI, the description is provided to indicate if wet, if blood or discharge was present, or any other pertinent description.

> **"4B) Site": The actual site is assessed by pulling back or removing the dressing.** As split gauze is used for this patient, it is simple to pull back parts to assess it. The skin is assessed to ensure there is no breakdown. The dressing is checked to see if any discharge (exudates) or bleeding was absorbed. The free-form line provides space to fully describe the site.

> **"4C) Care/TX": For this patient, the physician ordered**

**treatments to the site twice daily.** The dressing is removed and the bolster that holds the tube close to the skin is pulled back, allowing for full visualization. The site is then cleansed per physician orders. A water-resistant barrier, such as A+D ointment, is placed around the stoma for protection. It is then covered with a split-gauze dressing. Any and all care to the site is recorded to ensure the site remains intact and without inflammation or drainage.

> **"5) Stool":** **Bowel elimination, stool, for this patient is tracked using the "Bowel Elimination / Change Record."** However it is also captured here.

> **"5A) BM During Shift":** If the patient had a bowel movement during the shift, "Y" for "yes" would be circled. If none, "N" would be indicated.

> **"5B) Notes":** This is a free-form line provided to note information regarding bowel movements, whether suppositories or a laxative were administered, or any other information that specifically involves the patient's elimination pattern.

> **"6) Other":** This section provides alerts and information directly pertaining to a possible life-threatening situation because this patient has a trach. One of the biggest threats to a ventilator-dependent patient is aspiration, when food or fluids mixed with gastric acids and contents enter the lungs from the stomach via the esophagus. Once vomitus enters the mouth, there is potential of its entering the trachea. Trach patents are usually both

immuno-compromised and do not have a gag reflex that prohibits substances from entering the nearly sterile cavity of the lungs.

> **"6A) Nausea":** If the patient was nauseous during the shift, "Y" for "yes" is circled.

> **"6B) Emesis":** If the patient vomited during the shift, "Y" for "yes" is circled.

> **"6C) Other":** This free-form line could be used to indicate measures taken to eliminate any nausea. If the patient did vomit, the emesis could be described and/or actions taken could be indicated. The purpose of this line is to provide vital information concerning the possible risk of aspiration.

> **"7) Addl Info":** Space is available at the end of the section to highlight additional information that may be pertinent and specific to this system only, the patient's gastrointestinal functioning, for ease in capturing and reviewing.

- **GENITOURINARY: Daily care and assessment is essential, and this section is used to assess and detail urinary function and changes throughout the shift.**

> **"Time":** The actual time of the undergarment change is noted. This coincides with the time slated on the "Bowel Elimination / Change Record" form.

> **"Saturation":** The voided amount is determined

subjectively by the saturation. Descriptive terms include "heavy", "full," "moderate," and "minimal."

**> "Odor": As a first indicator of urinary tract infection,** changes to urine odor are noted. If odor is present, it is described as "mild," "strong," or "foul," for example. It must be stated, however, that urine odors present stronger depending on the time between undergarment (diaper) changes.

**> "Full Chg":** Typically a full disposable undergarment change is performed for this patient. This includes a new diaper, a new insert, and skin care. However, if it could not be performed, the insert only would be changed. If a full care was provided, then "Y" for "yes" would be circled. If a full change was not done, then "N" would be indicated.

**> "Insert":** If a full diaper change was performed, the insert would be removed and replaced. In those instances when a full change could not be performed, the nurse indicates the disposition of the insert. For this patient, an insert is always removed and replaced, minimally at pre-determined times.

**> "*) Addl Info":** Space is available at the end of the section to highlight additional information that may be pertinent and specific to this system only, the patient's genital or urinary functioning, for ease in capturing and reviewing.

- **MUSCULOSKETAL/SKIN: This section is used to assess and care for the muscles, bones and skin as well as doc-**

ument care to eliminate skin breakdown throughout the shift.

> "1) Description: The patient's skin is assessed for temperature, moisture, and color**. The appropriate descriptive phrase is circled. More than one could be circled; for example, a patient with a high fever could be assessed as being "hot" and "diaphoretic" (covered in sweat). "Color" indicates perfusion to the observable skin. In times of infection, the skin may be flushed or red. When perfusion is not adequate to fingers and toes, the tips may appear blue or with pallor. Color and any abnormalities are noted in this field.

> "2) Condition": The status, condition, and description of the patient's skin are noted here.** It focuses on any skin surface that is not intact. Descriptions and locations of breakdown are noted in this area comprised of three fields to detail problems such as bruises (ecchymosis), cuts, abrasions, non-blanchable areas, *etc.* Wound dressing and care should also be provided. This section is to promote healthy skin, enhance healing, and prevent or eliminate tissue breakdown.

> "2A) Intact":** This field provides quick reference whether there is current and active breakdown of the patient's skin. If there is a skin tear, a non-blanchable reddened area, or an open wound, for example, "N" for "no" would be circled. If the skin is intact, without any incidence of breakdown, "Y" is indicated.

> "2B) Dsg Locations & Types":** Any dressing used to

heal a wound is indicated along with the location of the body to which it is applied. Dressings could also be used proactively to protect an area that had previous breakdown.

> **"2C) Wound Descr"**: A description of any wound or healed wound that is currently being treated or protected by a dressing is described in the field. Additionally, any abnormality, such as bruises (ecchymoses) or other incidences such as a cut or bug bite, would also be noted in this area, even if not treated or dressed.

> **"2D) Tx"**: Any care given to actively treated or protected wound is described here. This includes any cleaning of the area, medication applications, and type of dressing used.

> **"3) Care"**: Cleaning the skin is performed throughout the day for sanitation and comfort. These fields provide information of the type of care performed during each nursing shift. Descriptions follow.

**Pericare** is an abbreviation for "perineum care". The perineum is the area between the vulva or scrotum, and the anus. During each undergarment change, the perineum is cleansed and dried fully. If pericare was performed during a shift, this is circled. If a full bed **bath** was provided during the shift, this is circled. When the patient's **hair** is **washed** during the shift, this is circled. **A+D** ointment is applied after pericare to the gluteal muscles to protect from wetness or stool. Additionally, after the cleaning of the PEG site, A+D is also applied to protect the skin from any discharge. If A+D was applied to any part of the body, those locations are noted here. **Lotion** is applied throughout the day to the back during under-garment changes and well as to the face and extremities. When and where it is applied is noted in this field.

> **"4) T&P On Right Side at (Time)": To maintain skin in-tegrity and minimize breakdown, the patient is turned from her back and placed on her right side periodically throughout the day**. In most cases, a patient would also be placed occasionally on the left side. However, this patient is unable to tolerate being on the left even for short durations. Only the full clock time the patient was placed on the right side is indicated here, for example 2:00-3:45 p.m... The amount of time is not used. When the patient is on her back, no time is indicated.

> **"5) OOB via Hoyer to WC": Daily, this patient gets out of bed (OOB) to a wheelchair (WC). This is accom-plished by using a Hoyer Lift.** The patient is placed on a sling. The sling is then attached to the lift, and mechani-cally she is raised up from the bed and positioned to be lowered into a wheelchair. If she was out of bed during the shift, "Y" for "yes" is circled. The amount of time she was out of bed, "Duration," is also noted.

> **"6) Pruritus":** At times the skin can become irritated, tingling, or itchy, and the need to scratch or rub the area is required to bring relief. This is pruritus. If the patient experienced this during the shift, "Y" for "yes" would be indicated. The area that was affected and any treatment, such as application of cream, is noted under "Area & Tx".

**> "7) PROM":** **Passive range of motion exercises are performed for this patient.** They are passive because the patient cannot actively move her joints. By providing range of motion movements overall, joint health is maintained. **These exercises are essential to limit contractures and maintain joint flexibility.**

**> "8) Addl Info":** Space is available at the end of the section to highlight additional information that may be pertinent and specific to this system only, the patient's muscle, skeletal and skin health and functioning, for ease in capturing and reviewing.

- **PSYCHO/SOCIAL: This section is used to assess and detail psycho-social well-being and changes throughout the shift.**

**> "1) Pt Concerns":** Any patient concerns, such as anxiety, worry, fear, sadness, uneasiness are noted. Conversely, positive feelings would also be documented, such as hope, faith, optimism or cheerfulness. The patient's concern may be about their health status but is not limited to this. Other aspects of the patient's life could also be included in this section, such as family or money issues, expectation of an anticipated visit, or any other non-health related subject.

**> "2) Sleep / Rest":** Sleep is vital to health and healing. This field documents the patient's sleep and either the clock time or the total amount of time could be provided. The amount of time slept is also important in evaluating the patient's mood or concerns.

> **"3) Mood / Disposition":** This provides a snap-shot of the patient's frame of mind. Entries are made at the **beginning** of the shift and the end of the shift. Short descriptive phrases are used such as "pleasant," "angry," "quiet," "sleepy," or "restless."

> **" 4) Addl Info":** Space is available at the end of the section to highlight additional information that may be pertinent and specific to this subject only, the patient's psychological and emotional well-being and changes, for ease in capturing and reviewing.

- **NOTES:** Although space is provided in each section to allow for free-form documentation, those lines are dedicated to the system in which they appear. This section of blank lines allow for additional documentation, or nursing notes, that may be related any topics. Blank lines and space allow the nurse to communicate anything deemed vital and important that occurred during the shift.

- **NURSE'S SIGNATURE:** The full legal signature and title of the nurse who performed the shift is completed here.

# EXHIBIT #8:
# BOWEL ELIMINATION / CHANGE RECORD

*Bowel Elimination / Change Record:* Page 1 (06/2015)

## Patient Name

| Name | For Month / Year | Prepared By | Date |
|---|---|---|---|

Perform full depends change q4h & PRN. Record bowel elimination w/brief
quantity ("amt") & quality ("qual") assessment per code

| | Time | 1 | 2 | 3 | 4 | 5 | 6 |
|---|---|---|---|---|---|---|---|
| | 12a | | | | | | |
| **AMT** | amt | | | | | | |
| small = S | qual | | | | | | |
| medium = M | 4a | | | | | | |
| large = L | amt | | | | | | |
| extra = X | qual | | | | | | |
| | 8a | | | | | | |
| | amt | | | | | | |
| **QUAL** | qual | | | | | | |
| formed = F | 12p | | | | | | |
| semi-formed = M | amt | | | | | | |
| loose = L | qual | | | | | | |
| hard = H | 4p | | | | | | |
| soft = S | amt | | | | | | |
| pasty = P | qual | | | | | | |
| diarrhea = D | 8p | | | | | | |
| runny = R | amt | | | | | | |
| smear = A | qual | | | | | | |
| ooze = Z | PRN | | | | | | |
| | amt | | | | | | |
| | qual | | | | | | |
| | PRN | | | | | | |
| | amt | | | | | | |
| | qual | | | | | | |

| Nurse's Signature | | Initials | Nurse's Signature |
|---|---|---|---|
| | | | |
| | | | |

## FIELD DESCRIPTIONS FOR BOWEL ELIMINATION / CHANGE RECORD

**This two-sided form is merely a table. Completion requires only the nurse's initials and use of a code to quantify and qualify the patient's stool.** The first line indicates the patient name, month, and the individual that prepared the form. The next line provides treatment specifics and form completion instructions. The remaining fields on the form are detailed below:

**First Vertical Column:** This provides the time frame for undergarment changes, for example every 4 hours (q4h). Also provided are codes to describe quantity and quality of any stool.

**Second Vertical Column:** Each undergarment change time frame is divided into a three-part section. The first line in each section is the **time** when changes are scheduled. The subsequent two lines below describe the amount ("**amt**") and quality ("**qual**") of the stool in each time segment.

**> TIME:** The time the undergarment change should occur is noted here. This is preset. The nurse or caregiver initials that it was completed in this field.

**> "AMT":** This is the amount of stool present during that particular undergarment change. To indicate the bowel movement size, codes from column one are used due to size limitations of the field. If the amount was extra-large, for example, we use "XL". Zeros, in this field and the next, indicate a lack of bowel elimination.

**> "QUAL":** This field describes the quality of the stool. There are many ways to describe stool, especially in a patient who is immobile and obtaining all nutrition from a liquid source. More than one code could be used each time. For example, stool could be soft and pasty, formed and hard, or formed and soft. Again, codes are used for lack of descriptive space.

**If additional detail of output is necessary, space is provided on the Nursing Review / Assessment Sheet.** Although not seen in nursing textbooks, it is not unusual to compare stool consistency to foods. Using this can eliminate personal variances in descriptions. For example, the consistency of mashed potatoes versus pudding yield two different textures although very similar—one more formed than the other. Rocks are not the same as grapes—both formed but certainly different in pliability.

> **Remaining Vertical Columns:** Each is numbered from 1 to 31 of this two-sided document. The number depicts the day of the month.

> **"NURSE'S SIGNATURE/INITIALS"**: A signature box follows last to identify all nurses that provided care that month. After the signature, each provides initials which are then used to identify the responsible professional who completed, assessed, and documented the action.

# EXHIBIT #9:
# RX MEDICATION TRANSLATION

## RX MEDICATION TRANSLATION (02/2016)

### DAILY MEDICATIONS

| BRAND | GENERIC | | GENERIC | BRAND |
|---|---|---|---|---|
| Ativan.................lorazepam | | | amlodipine..............Norvasc | |
| *Anti-anxiety, sedative* | | | *Anti-hypertensive; Ca²⁺ Channel Blocker* | |
| Baclofen..............lioresal | | | duloxetine HCl.........Cymbalta | |
| *Anti-spasticity, Skeletal muscle relaxant* | | | *Anti-depressant; SSRNI* | |
| Carafate..............sucralfate | | | fluoxetine HCl..........Prozac | |
| *Anti-ulcer; GI protectant* | | | *Anti-depressant; SSRI* | |
| Cymbalta.............duloxetine HCl | | | lioresal.....................Baclofen | |
| *Anti-depressant; SSRNI* | | | *Anti-spasticity,  Skeletal muscle relaxant* | |
| Elocon.................mometasone cream | | | lorazepam...............Ativan | |
| *Topical corticosteroid* | | | *Anti-anxiety, sedative* | |
| Klor-Con KCl........potassium chloride | | | mometasone............Elocon | |
| *Electrolyte replacement/supplement* | | | *Topical corticosteroid* | |
| Macrodantin........nitrofurantoin | | | nitrofurantoin..........Macrodantin | |
| *Anti-infective; UTI prophylactic* | | | *Anti-infective; UTI prophylactic* | |
| Norvasc................amlodipine besylate | | | potassium CL............Klor-Con KCl | |
| *Anti-hypertensive; Calcium channel blocker* | | | *Electrolyte supplement* | |
| Prozac...................fluoxetine HCl | | | sucralfate.................Carafate | |
| *Anti-depressant; SSRI* | | | *Anti-ulcer; GI protectant* | |

### PRN MEDICATIONS

| BRAND | GENERIC | | GENERIC | BRAND |
|---|---|---|---|---|
| Ativan.................lorazepam | | | clobestasol...............Clobex | |
| *Anti-anxiety, sedative; Benzodiazephine* | | | *Enzymatic debrider* | |
| Bactroban Oint...mupirocin | | | collagenase...............Santyl Oint | |
| *Anti-infective* | | | *Topical sulfa antibiotic* | |
| Clobex (eg).........clobetasol propionate | | | desoximetasone.......Topicort | |
| *High potency topical corticosteroid* | | | *Topical corticosteroid* | |
| Halcion.................triazolam | | | lorazepam.................Ativan | |
| *Sedative; Benzodiazepines* | | | *Anti-anxiety, sedative* | |
| Morphine...........morphine sulfate | | | morphine sulfate.....Morphine | |
| *Opiod analgesic* | | | *Opiod analgesic* | |
| Nasacort..............trimcinolone | | | mupirocin.................Bactroban Oint | |
| *Corticosteroid nasal spray* | | | *Anti-infective* | |
| Santyl Oint...........collagenase | | | silver sulphadiazine....Silvadene | |
| *Topical sulfa antibiotic* | | | *Enzymatic debrider* | |
| Silvadene.............silver sulphadiazine | | | triazolam....................Halcion | |
| *Enzymatic debrider* | | | *Sedative; Benzodiazepines* | |
| Topicort ..............desoximetasone | | | trimcinolone.............Nasacort | |
| *Topical corticosteroid* | | | *Corticosteroid nasal spray* | |

**EXHIBIT #9:** Field Descriptions for **RX** Medication Translation

Medications can be dispensed in either generic or brand substances depending on the pharmacy, insurance, or even the availability of the medication at the pharmacy when the prescription is filled. To aid nursing staff and family members, we utilize a Pharmacy (RX) Medication Translation Record. This document provides an alphabetical listing of the brand and generic names of all medications that this patient is or may be given in the course of a day. Specific details follow.

> Medications are separated according to administrations. Daily meds are noted in the first section. The second portion lists all medications that can be administered on an "as needed basis" ("PRN").

> Whether daily or PRN medication, the first vertical grouping provides the **"BRAND"** name of the drug in alphabetical order. The generic translation for that specific brand then follows to the right. Immediately under the drug, the purpose for the administration of that medication is provided.

> The second vertical grouping performs in a similar way as the "BRAND" grouping discussed above. The difference, however, is that this section list the medications alphabetically according the **"GENERIC"** name. Immediately next to the generic name, the brand name translation is provided. Again, under the drug, the medication's purpose is noted.

www.ingramcontent.com/pod-product-compliance
Lightning Source LLC
Chambersburg PA
CBHW051439170526
45166CB00001B/40